FIGHTERS OF FATE

FIGHTERS OF FATE

*A STORY OF MEN AND
WOMEN WHO HAVE ACHIEVED GREATLY
DESPITE THE HANDICAPS OF THE
GREAT WHITE PLAGUE*

BY

JAY ARTHUR MYERS

WITH AN INTRODUCTION BY

CHARLES H. MAYO

Essay Index Reprint Series

BOOKS FOR LIBRARIES PRESS
FREEPORT, NEW YORK

First Published 1927
Reprinted 1969

STANDARD BOOK NUMBER:
8369-1099-0

LIBRARY OF CONGRESS CATALOG CARD NUMBER:
79-84329

PRINTED IN THE UNITED STATES OF AMERICA

TO THE MEMORY OF MY MOTHER

a continuing benediction,—in grateful apprecia-tion of the much she helped her son, of the stimulus she always gave to his highest possibili-ties of achievement, of her constant urge to faith-ful service, this book, with deep reverence and tenderness, is dedicated.

CONTENTS

INTRODUCTION

CONTEMPORARY history is always superficial because it can record, at the best, mere facts and events. Not until the actors have passed from the stage can the historian dissect the past, and expose the ambitions and passions and the medley of strength and weakness, of altruism and vanity, of love and hate, that moved the wheels of history. Not until the marionettes have lost their contact with the present does he dare to follow the French advice, *cherchez la femme*, and discover the woman's hand that often pulled the strings. In this book, the author has carried analysis one step further: his motto is *"cherchez le microbe."*

Of the famous men and those who contributed largely to the advancement of science, literature, art and music, he has been able to point to a surprisingly large number who were victims of tuberculosis. While his list might be greatly amplified, the proportion of great men among the tuberculous is probably no greater than among the nontuberculous. Statistical studies are out of the question, and the subject is not approached from that angle. Moreover, there is no certainty about the diagnosis. Chronic cough and general poor health were considered marks of "a decline" even a generation ago. Even our present day enlightenment does not prevent the sanitoriums from harboring a very considerable percentage of unconvicted suspects; and the errors of the general practitioner must be still greater. The more remote the historical character, the less authentic is the history of tuberculosis.

The author wishes to encourage and stimulate the stricken by the example of those who not only held up their heads under the blow, but actually turned misfortune to their own betterment.

The success of the individual depends largely on heredity, opportunity, environment and education. The seeds of great mental achievement may be dormant for generations and only sprout when change of environment provides the opportunity. The seed may be uprooted from unfriendly soil only by the prongs of apparent misfortune. The weakling may find in sheltered occupation the sun that warms his dormant faculties to life. The artisan, shorn of his strength, may only then learn that his brain is far mightier than his hands. Tuberculosis is very often the fruit of an undisciplined and rebellious state of mind. The ne'er-do-well and the drifter are pulled up short by fear and learn their first lesson in the remorselessness of law. The years spent in voluntary obedience to the rules of treatment may have a lasting influence and remove the one great obstacle to success in life.

Many poisons have a stimulating effect on mental processes. Alcohol is produced by a microbe; morphine, belladonna and cocaine are products of vegetable cells. Intoxication in the usual sense often accompanies intoxication in the medical sense. Almost any infection may produce delirium, which is mental stimulation carried to its extreme. As with these intoxicating drugs, there should be a point at which the effect would be no more than exaltation, and those microbic poisons which produce only a slow effect might be expected to stop at the stage of mild stimulation. We know that victims of chronic tuberculosis have learned the significance of the feeling of unusual vitality and vigor that often precedes increase in cough, slight fever and another bout with the enemy. Man is not the only creature whom Nature has cunningly equipped for the struggle of life; the little speck of living matter known as the bacillus of tuberculosis paves the way for its destructive action by stimulating its host to over-activity. Like the Roman gods, whom it seeks to destroy, it first makes mad.

There are other microbes which have a depressing effect, notably those which affect the colon. Instead of considering the effect of the stars and moon on character and conduct, we now study, in a rather speculative way, the endocrine glands and the intestinal flora. To those who are unable to encompass the conception of two co-existing causes, ethics is merely one of the offshoots of bacteriology. Modern surgery could have recast one of Shakespeare's most famous characters, and "Hamlet" might have ended in the banquet-hall instead of the grave-yard. Shakespeare himself would thus owe his versatility to a menagerie of microbes which he exhibited in turn.

Dr. Myers indulges in none of these speculations. He merely parades before our eyes men who denied adversity its toll and used misfortune as a stepping-stone. Let us not quibble while his heroes speak.

CHARLES H. MAYO, M.D.

Rochester, Minn.
   April 1926.

FOREWORD

THERE are those who state that tuberculosis is never healed, that its victims are never able to do anything worth while after the development of this disease. There are still others who believe that the tuberculous patient is not capable of accomplishment while the disease exists. Frequently encountering these arguments, I have decided to compile facts regarding the lives of a few of the world's outstanding characters who have suffered from tuberculosis, in the hope that these facts will suffice for all time to prove that the tuberculous patient is worth saving, that tuberculosis does heal, and that the tuberculous patient is often capable of great accomplishments.

There is a kinship in tuberculosis that is unique, as Eugene O'Neill points out. The types of experience gained in battling tuberculosis are peculiar to that disease alone. Hence the lives of other tuberculous individuals have a deeper significance to the sufferer from tuberculosis. The comparison of the accomplishments of the average individual with those of a tuberculous patient would be unfair, yet the accomplishments of other tuberculous individuals is a proper criterion.

In the present collection the lives are selected in order to be far more than a standard or measure. Their purpose is to provide an incentive or stimulus to the recovered or recovering patient to start life anew and most of all to prove to the suffering patient that all is not lost because he is temporarily overpowered by tuberculosis.

The scope of the subject matter is wide both in time and location, for the inroads of tuberculosis are universal and almost prehistoric. The achievements of persons who lived before the bulk of the modern conception of tuberculosis and its treatment was accumulated take on the proportions of heroic attainments. They had to fight their own disease, public opinion and prejudice, and almost Nature herself. Today the patient works with Nature and Science to conquer his disease and in an enlightened world that offers an equal opportunity for success to the tuberculous as well as the nontuberculous. The former situation is most clearly shown by the life of Paganini, while the latter is demonstrated by the life of Babson. Which condition is better is self-evident.

The problems and solutions of the subjects of these sketches while not identical with those of every patient are still analagous enough to prove that there is a way out of every difficulty that is compatible with the special considerations imposed by the disease. This may mean the altering of an ambition or the modification of the mode of life but it does not imply a life of invalidism or dependence on others.

The accomplishments of tuberculous patients cited will be of interest to the general public not only because they illustrate success but also because they illustrate that failure is not synonymous with a breakdown from tuberculosis. The following sketches prove conclusively that every effort possible should bend toward the saving of the tuberculous, for they will be saved to make some contribution to the lives of others and perhaps this contribution will be an invaluable one for the world. All tuberculosis workers, as well as the patients themselves, cannot but be heartened by the facts included in these various lives.

Havelock Ellis, in "A Study of British Genius" has pointed out that tuberculosis was present in at least forty British personages, each of them a genius. What is true of British genius is no doubt true for the most part of genius of other nations. Tuberculosis does not produce genius, however. The life of physical inactivity which the tuberculous patient is frequently compelled to live may give him an opportunity to discover or develop his native powers. Such is the case of Eugene O'Neill. Tuberculosis is accredited with causing a mental exaltation and increased excitability during which great visions and plans for their realization come to the patient. Chopin is said to have been motivated in the composition of some of his masterpieces by such a condition. In some measure this may be true, but the greater opportunities for increased mental activity as a result of the decreased physical capacity account for most of the relationship between tuberculosis and genius.

Tuberculous foci may be healed, but not always, nor for all time. Recovery from tuberculosis depends on a number of factors, and in the absence of any of these essential conditions persons will die of the disease. If any of these factors of safety are lacking they may be developed before the disease has destroyed too much of the vital tissue of the body. So much has been learned about these necessary factors in combating tuberculosis that the plague has been greatly controlled in the past few years. In certain communities over four hundred persons died of this disease in 1820, where in 1920, less than one hundred died. In this group of people in whom not all the essential factors of complete healing can be developed, the disease is held in abeyance. Its host, although not always up to par, is capable of doing considerable work and living out the natural span of human life.

Many persons possess most of the factors necessary to healing at the onset of the attack. Some with no special aid and others with but slight assistance make excellent recoveries. A striking example of this is to be found in the history of Elizabeth Barrett Browning. Such persons suffer initially from unmistakable tuberculosis of the lungs; but with healing of the disease they may resume their heavy tasks and may greatly enrich the world by their subsequent contributions; finally dying of conditions other than those of tuberculosis. Tuberculosis heals completely in the human body as well as in animals. The evidence frequently revealed at post mortem examinations of tuberculous processes fully healed found in the bodies of men and women who died of other causes, is irrefutable.

Since the discovery of the tubercle bacillus in 1882 by Koch, constructive measure for prevention and cure of tuberculosis have been developed and the knowledge of them disseminated through

the world. Although no definite specific has
come into accepted use, the general measures of
rest, good food, good ventilation, and medical
and nursing supervision have been applied pro-
portionally to their relative values. Mechanical
devices have been perfected which increase the
amount of rest possible to a diseased lung. Sana-
toria have been built and equipped for the hos-
pitalization of the tuberculous and preventive
regulations for the protection of the public have
been commonly applied.

To sum it all up, the tuberculous patient of
today and the people at large have superior and
more readily available opportunities of health
recovery and health preservation than the race
has enjoyed since the very beginning of time.

And not only is it possible to regain one's
health, but also to regain one's former status in
life. This is, in itself, a thing worth striving for.
Leadership in literature, art, music, business or
professional service is not attainable by everyone.
The value of a life is not measured by fortune or
by education or by attendance upon a formal institution of learning, any more than is its worth to
others determined by the extent of worldly fame.
Every patient, potential genius has the world
before him in which to live a life of usefulness
and honor, despite the handicap of tuberculosis.

FOREWORD

The selection of these life stories has been difficult, since there is available so large a number of worthy ones. There are many others, and of no less importance, whose lives I had strongly desired to include, but whose addition to the list would have added unduly to the length of the work. An extended study of the references will delight the interested reader.

To the following who so kindly and generously have helped me in the preparation of this volume, I wish to express my deep appreciation: President Lotus D. Coffman, Rev. Roy L. Smith, Superintendent W. F. Webster, Dr. E. R. Baldwin, Dr. A. K. Krause, Dr. Philip P. Jacobs, Dr. H. S. Diehl, Dr. R. E. Scammon, Dr. H. Longstreet Taylor, Dr. E. A. Meyerding, Dr. R. O. Beard, Miss Beatrice Tomelty, Miss Edith Corson, Mrs. Hazel Garland, Mr. Alfred Green, Miss Blanche Boquist and Miss Nancy Leach. I am deeply indebted to the relatives of some subjects of my study, of recent passing, and to some who still living have kindly aided me in the compilation of data.

J. A. M.

NICOLO PAGANINI

NICOLO PAGANINI was born at Genoa,
Italy, on October 27, 1782, instead of in
1784, as was formerly believed. His father
was a shopkeeper, a greedy and covetous person
who saw in his son's genius only a means of
gaining money. The family lived in a squalid
neighborhood by the harbor occupied by the
poorest people of Genoa. Nicolo had two sisters
and one brother. Concerning the lives of the
sisters, nothing seems to be known, but the
brother is believed to have become a physician.

In early childhood, Nicolo had a severe attack
of measles, so severe that he was believed to be
dead. He was wrapped in a shroud, but just
before he was to be buried his body was seen to
move slightly and this evidence of life saved him
from being buried alive. As soon as he had
recovered sufficiently, his father began to give
him instruction on the violin. Nicolo showed
so much talent, though only a child, that his
father became very greedy of his future. He
could see a great fortune ahead of him and,
therefore, insisted that Nicolo work on his violin
lessons from early in the morning until late at

night. The father severely punished him for
any slight mistakes, even to the extent of beating him and withholding his food. Through all
this the mother, a lovable woman, by her kindness no doubt saved him from discouragement
and a hatred of his art. She told Nicolo of a
wonderful dream she had had. In this dream
an angel had promised to bring to pass any wish
of hers. She requested that Nicolo be allowed
to become the greatest of all violinists. The
angel promised to fulfill her desire.

When Nicolo had reached the age of six years,
he played so well that the neighbors were amazed,
indeed he was spoken of as "the wonder-child."
Already his attainments were so great that his
father could no longer teach him; so for a short
time, he became the pupil of Giovanni Servetto,
then the best violinist in Genoa. Giacoma Costa
took him as a pupil, with the understanding that
Nicolo would prepare and play, in one of the
churches, a new concerto each week. Because
of the close supervision which his father continued to exercise over him, Nicolo had no opportunity to enjoy games or to indulge in the
pleasures of childhood with other children.
Nevertheless, he developed rapidly and at the
age of eight years had composed a sonata for the
violin; while at the age of eleven years he played,

upon an occasion of prime importance, in the Great Theater of Genoa. In this performance he met with the greatest success.

Nicolo had so outgrown the musicians of Genoa that, when he was thirteen years old, on the recommendation of his former teacher, Costa, he was taken to Parma where he was to be placed under Allessandro Rolla, the "Pride of Italy." Upon the arrival of Nicolo and his father, Rolla was ill and was not inclined to see visitors. In the room where Nicolo and his father were waiting was a violin and one of Rolla's compositions. Upon his father's insistence, Nicolo played the composition. Rolla, hearing it from his sick room, inquired as to what *virtuoso* was there. He would not believe that a boy of only thirteen years was responsible, until the performance had been repeated before his eyes. After this, he told Nicolo's father that the boy was beyond him and that he should be taken to Ferdinando Paer for instruction in composition. There is some evidence, however, to show that Nicolo later took some lessons with Rolla and that he did not remain long with Paer. The teacher who taught him most, in Parma, was Gasparo Ghiretti, who gave him careful work in composition and counterpoint.

In 1797, the boy was taken by his father on a

[3]

tour, during which he gave concerts in Pisa, Florence, Milan, Leghorn and Bologna. These concerts were splendidly received, but the father took entire charge of the financial returns. After reaching home, Nicolo continued to work, under the very strict supervision of his father, but it seems that his supervision applied only to music, for the boy's general education was entirely neglected. This was also true of his moral development. As time passed he grew more and more resentful toward his father because of his cruel treatment. At the age of seventeen with the aid of his mother he was allowed to leave home. He started out in the world with almost no equipment for life's battle except expertness in an art which would guarantee him a good financial income. It has been said that "Paganini's was a nature warped; on the one side phenomenal powers; on the other bodily suffering and intellectual and spiritual atrophy."

Upon leaving home, Paganini went to Lucca, then to Pisa and to many other places, where he gave concerts. He was earning a good living and was so glad to be free from his father's domination that he decided never to return home again. The future looked bright, but he selected the wrong kind of companions. Because of his

total lack of general education and moral training, as well as his present good earning ability
he was easy prey for the parasites of society. He
began to gamble. Of this period, Stratton
says: "Soon his talent provided fresh resources
and his days ran on in alternations of good and
evil fortune. Tall, slight, delicate, and handsome, Paganini, despite his frail constitution, was
an object of attraction to the fair sex. Incidents
in his early manhood probably formed the
foundation for some of the stories told of him
later. As Fetis puts it: the enthusiasm for art,
love, and 'play,' reigned by turns in his soul.
He ought to have been careful of himself, but
he went to excess in everything."

He became so confirmed a gambler that frequently he would lose the earnings of several
concerts at a single sitting. He had to dispose
of his violin in order to pay his honest debts.
On one occasion by gambling, he lost his violin,
just before he was to give a concert at Leghorn.
It appeared that he would be unable to fulfill
the engagement, but just in time he found it
possible to borrow a splendid Guarnerius of a
French merchant, who was an amateur violinist
and very enthusiastic over music. Upon Nicolo's
return of the instrument, the merchant said:
"I shall take care never to profane the strings

[5]

your fingers have touched. It is to you now that my violin belongs." This gift did much for Paganini. It broke his gambling habit, as later evidenced by his own statement. He wrote: "I shall never forget one day placing myself in a position which was to decide my whole career. The Prince De —— had long desired to possess my excellent violin, the Guarnerius, the only one I then had, and which I still possess. One day he desired me to fix a price; but, unwilling to part from my instrument, I declared I would not sell it for less than 250 gold Napoleons. A short time after, the Prince remarked that I was probably indulging in banter in asking so high a price, and added that he was disposed to give 2,000 francs for it. Precisely that very day I found myself in great want of money, in consequence of a heavy loss at play; and I almost resolved to yield my violin for the sum he had offered, when a friend came in to invite me to a party that evening. My capital then consisted of thirty francs, and I had already deprived myself of my jewels, watch, rings, pins, etc. I instantly formed the resolve to risk this last resource and, if fortune went against me, to sell the violin and to set out for St. Petersburg, without instrument and without funds, with the object of retrieving my position.

Soon my thirty francs were reduced to three, and I saw myself on the road to the great city, when fortune, changing in the twinkling of an eye, gained me one hundred francs with the little that yet remained. That moment saved my violin and set me up again. From that day I withdrew from play, to which I had sacrificed a portion of my youth; and, convinced that a gambler is universally despised, I renounced forever that fatal passion."

When Napoleon crossed the Alps and great turmoil reigned, Paganini disappeared from public view for over three years. He spent this time "at the chateau of a Tuscan lady of rank, who was a performer upon the guitar." Here he became as expert upon the guitar as upon the violin and composed music for both instruments. At this time he also made a rather intensive study of agriculture.

After Napoleon had parceled out Europe to his brothers and sisters and Italy was settled under the French government, in 1804, Paganini returned and, in 1805, was again giving his famous concerts. When he played at Lucca, the princess, a sister of Napoleon, offered to make him leader of the Court orchestra, and solo violinist. He accepted this position and while holding it he introduced the use of less than four

strings on the violin, which he describes thus:
"It fell to my lot," he said, "to direct the opera
whenever the reigning family visited it, as well
as to perform at Court, three times a week, and
to get up a public concert for the higher circles
every fortnight. Whenever these were visited
by the Princess she never remained to the close,
because the flageolet tones of my violin were too
much for her nerves. On the other hand there
was another fascinating creature . . . who,
I flattered myself, felt a penchant for me, and
was never absent from my performances; on my
own side, I had long been her admirer, [Paganini
was now twenty-three years of age, susceptible,
and, possibly, himself fascinating]. Our mutual
fondness became gradually stronger and stronger;
but we were forced to conceal it, and by this
means its strength and fervour were sensibly
enhanced. One day I promised to surprise her,
at the next concert, with a musical joke which
should convey an allusion to our attachment;
and I, accordingly, gave notice at Court that I
should bring forward a musical novelty, under
the title of 'A Love Scene.' The whole world
was on tiptoe at the tidings; and, on the evening
appointed, I made my appearance violin in hand.
I had previously robbed it of the two middle
strings, so that none but E and G remained.

[8]

The first string being designed to play the maiden's part, and the second (fourth) the youth's, I began with a species of dialogue, in which I attempted to introduce movements analogous to transient bickerings and reconciliations between the lovers. Now my strings growled, and then sighed, and anon they lisped, hesitated, joked and joyed,—till at last they sported with merry jubilee. In the course of time, both souls joined once more in harmony, and the appeased lover's quarrel led to a *pas de deux*, which terminated in a brilliant coda. This musical fantasia of mine was greeted with loud applause. The lady, to whom every scene referred, rewarded me by looks full of delight and sweetness; and the Princess was charmed into such amiable condescension, that she loaded me with enconiums,—asking me, whether, since I could produce so much with two strings, it would not be possible for me to gratify them by playing on one. I yielded instant assent—the idea tickled my fancy,—and, as the Emperor's birthday occurred some weeks afterwards [August 15th], I composed a sonata for the G string, which I entitled 'Napoleon' and played before the Court to so much effect, that a cantata, by Cimarosa, given the same evening, fell through without producing any impression on its hearers.

This is the genuine and original cause of my prejudice in favor of the G string. People were afterwards importunate to hear more of this performance, and in this way I became day by day a great adept at it, and acquired constantly increasing confidence in this peculiar mystery of handling the bow."

The experiment served, however, to relieve him of considerable embarrassment three years later. Just before he was to give a concert at Leghorn, he ran a nail into his heel which caused him to come on the stage limping. The amusement of the audience was evidenced by its facial expressions, which Paganini did not fail to observe. As he was beginning to play, the candles toppled from the music stand. When the laughter ceased and he had barely begun to play again, one of his violin strings broke. Although he was sensitive and the laughter was uproarous, he completely won the audience by continuing and finishing the concert with the three remaining strings of the violin.

In 1813, Paganini resigned his official position. Then he was free to make many tours. He spent much time, during the coming year, giving concerts in the Italian cities. In 1826, the same year as Laennec died, Paganini visited Rome and, in the following year, Pope Leo XII invested him with the order of the Golden Spur. Having traveled throughout his homeland so many times, he decided to go to "Musical Vienna" in 1828. Here as in his own country he was splendidly received, as evidenced by this comment: "At the first stroke of the bow on his Guarnerius, one might almost say at the first step he took into the hall, his reputation in Germany was decided. Kindled as by an electric flash, he suddenly shone and sparkled like a miraculous apparition in the domain of art."

So successful were Paganini's concerts in Vienna that it was found necessary to double the number originally scheduled. No halls could be found large enough to contain all who wished to hear him. Poor musicians are said to have sold some of their clothing to obtain enough money to gain admission. In Vienna, however, while playing "The Witch's Dance," a member of the audience claimed to have seen the devil, with horns, a tail, and dressed in red, appear by the side of Paganini and direct his actions. Thus was noised about Vienna that Paganini was supposed to be in league with the devil. Stratton points out that, at that time, the devil was regarded as a real personage and that the uneducated had already been taught to associate the violin with the devil, because of the story of Tartini and his dreams. To us such an incident seems absurd; but, nevertheless, it was believed by the more ignorant and superstitious among the people and was ever after used to great advantage by Paganini's enemies.

At another time, a rumor became extant that Paganini had spent eight years in prison as a punishment for murder. Those who spread this rumor insisted that his great skill was due to the fact that while in prison he had nothing to do but practice upon the violin. Even pictures were made representing him in prison. Although there was not one word of truth in this rumor, it, too, was believed by many and was used persistently by his enemies.

From Vienna, Paganini, later went to Prague, Berlin, Leipzig and other cities. While in Hamburg, the great German poet, Heine, heard Paganini. Heine said: "I believe that only one man has succeeded in putting Paganini's true physiognomy upon paper, a deaf painter, Lyser by name, who in a frenzy of genius has with a few strokes of chalk so well hit the great violinist's head that one is at the same time amused and terrified at the truth of the drawing. 'The devil guided my hand' the deaf painter said to me, chuckling mysteriously, and nodding his head with a good-natured irony in the way he generally accompanied his genial witticisms. The Hamburg Opera House was the scene of this concert, and the art-loving public had flocked there so early, and in such numbers, that I only just succeeded in obtaining a little place in the orchestra. Is that a man, brought into the arena at the moment of death, like a dying gladiator, to delight the public with his convulsions? Or is it one risen from the dead, a vampire with a violin, who, if not the blood out of our hearts, at any rate sucks the gold out of our pockets? Such questions crossed our minds while Paganini was performing his strange bows, but all these thoughts were at once stilled when the wonderful master placed his violin under his chin and began to play. As for me, you already know my musical second-sight, my gift of seeing at each tone a figure equivalent to the sound, and so Paganini with each stroke of his bow brought visible forms and situations before my eyes; he told me in melodious hieroglyphics all kinds of brilliant tales; he as it were, made a magic lantern play its colored antics before me, he himself being the chief actor. A holy, ineffable ardor dwelt in the sounds, which often trembled, scarce audibly, in mysterious whisper on the water; then swelled out again with a shuddering sweetness, like a bugle's notes heard by moonlight, and then finally poured forth in unrestrained jubilee, as if a thousand hands had struck their harps and raised their voices in a song of victory."

In 1829, Paganini played in Warsaw. There Chopin heard him and was inspired by him. Upon departing from Warsaw, Joseph Elsener, Chopin's teacher, presented Paganini with an expensive snuff box.

After having been splendidly received in Paris, Paganini left for London, in May, 1831. Although considerable criticism of his coming had appeared in the London papers a musician and critic wrote, regarding his first performance, as follows: "The long, laboured, reiterated articles relative to Paganini, in all the foreign journals for years past, have spoken of his power as so astonishing, that we were quite prepared to find them fall far short of report; but his performances at his first concert, on the third of last month, convinced us that it is possible to exceed the most sanguine expectations and to surpass what the most eulogistic writers have asserted. We speak, however, let it be understood, in reference to his powers of execution solely. These are little less than marvelous, and such as we could only have believed on the evidence of our own senses. They imply a strong natural pro-

pensity to music, with an industry, a perseverance, a devotedness, and also a skill in inventing
means without any parallel in the history of
his instrument."

After giving up gambling Paganini spent his
money wisely so that upon his return to Italy in
1834, after six years of touring in foreign countries,
he was rich. He bought a great deal of land,
including a beautiful home near Parma.

In 1824, after recovering from a serious illness,
at Genoa, two girls aided Paganini in giving a
concert. One of them, Signora Bionchi, sang
three songs, while the other performed on the
violoncello. Signora Bionchi became Paganini's
companion and while he was giving his concerts
in Vienna his son was born. Later, when they
went to England, apparently because of Signora
Bionchi's jealous temper, Paganini separated
from her, and fell in love with the daughter of the
man in whose house he lodged. This young lady
had taken part in some of Paganini's concerts
and she, too, had fallen deeply in love with him.
They arranged to be married in Paris. Paganini
was to leave and the young lady was to meet
him in Boulogne later. This was all to be
carried out in secret. The young lady, in due
time, left her home; but her father, suspicious of
her whereabouts, hurried to Boulogne and when

she arrived, he, instead of Paganini, met her. The father and the daughter immediately journeyed home together. Later, this young lady came to America as an actress and it is said that Paganini sent a special agent to interview her, but they never married.

Paganini's health was broken when he was a mere child, under the brutal treatment of his father. When only sixteen years old, in 1798, he was terribly dissipated. Not infrequently, because of his absolute exhaustion, he was forced to discontinue his activities for weeks at a time. Unfortunately, as soon as he was well rested, he would again resort to the expenditure of his energies at a fearful rate. In 1819, the year Laennec published his first book on the stethoscope, Paganini's health had so completely broken down that his landlord made a diagnosis of consumption. He was living in Naples and, because in that place there was so strong a belief that consumption was contagious, the landlord threw Paganini and his equipment into the street. Ciandelli, a friend, was passing by and saw the episode. He was not convinced of the contagiousness of consumption and certainly did not approve of this form of open air treatment; consequently he gave the landlord a sound beating. This being well done, he found good quarters and excellent care elsewhere for the tuberculous violinist.

Paganini made a temporary recovery and, later continued with his work, only to break down again, in 1823, while on his way to Pavia. This time he became so ill that it was believed he could not make even a temporary recovery; nevertheless, after a long period of rest in Genoa, he was again able to give his concerts. In the matter of food, also, his health had not been sufficiently guarded, for it is said that often he would have only a cup of chocolate for breakfast and take no more food until night. This was particularly true when he was making long journeys. In 1828, while in Vienna, it has been said: "He was in his forty-sixth year and his face bore the marks of suffering; he wore his long hair in ringlets falling over his shoulders, but physically he was a wreck." Upon finishing his engagements in Vienna he was prostrated, so he repaired to Carlsbad for a period of rest. When, later, he went to Prague he developed an abscess on his face which finally led to an operation on the jaw-bone. By 1834, when he returned to Italy, after six years spent in touring other countries, his health was in a desperate state. Not only did he have advanced tuberculosis of the lungs, but he also had tuberculosis of the larynx or voice organ, so that he found it difficult to speak. The next year he spent most of his time in Genoa, Milan and about Parma. He apparently took good care of his health, for in 1837 he had so far improved as to be able to give several concerts. During the next year, he seemed to have continued to improve, "for the papers spoke of his becoming corpulent." By 1839, he was ill again and sought benefit in climatic change. In later years, he insisted upon having the windows of the carriage in which he was riding closed, but upon arrival in his rooms he threw the windows wide open and took frequent sun-baths. Each new climate seemed to be all that was necessary to restore his health, but as its newness "wore off" he found himself no better. Thus he continued to change climates, all the time actually growing worse, but, truly characteristic of the consumptive, always grasping with out-stretched arms for every fragment of the floating driftwood of hope. He died on May 27, 1840. His body was buried in the Communal Cemetery at the Villa Cajona. In 1888, the body was exhumed and reinterred in the Central Cemetery at Vienna.

Perhaps because of the cruel treatment Paganini suffered as a child, he did all he could to protect his own son. It has been said that he "became avaricious," but it was for the sake of his little boy, whose life he desired might be better than his own. "He saves for his yet un- educated child," wrote Guhr, in 1829, "Yes, this man, proud, scornful, despising the crowds whose money made him rich, in the recesses of his heart nourished a love, pure and unselfish. That was the fine gold; his wealth was dross. His affection for the child was boundless and he allowed the little fellow to tyrannize over him completely. There are rare pretty stories of his playing with the boy, but there is nothing about teaching the boy to play the violin. The memory of his own childhood was quite sufficient to deter him from any attempt to force instruction on his boy and to cloud the sunshine of his young life."

Paganini gave many concerts for the benefit of the poor in the great cities he visited. One day he encountered a small Italian boy playing on the street in Vienna. The boy said that his mother was ill and that he had to beg to support her. Paganini not only gave the boy all the money he had with him, but took out his violin and began to play. Soon a large crowd gathered around to hear the unknown master violinist. Then he took up a collection, which was liberal. He turned it over to the boy and said: "Take that to your mother." Many similar incidents are on record to prove the good-heartedness of the great musician.

In summing up the value of Paganini's life to the world and the world's appreciation of it, Stratton says: "Such outward honors as the world gives to its dead have indeed been offered to the memory of Paganini; but it is doubtful whether the higher honor of a frank recognition by the musical world of the work that he did for it has ever been his. Unlike the great composer, the instrumentalist leaves behind him no visible proof of the part he has played in the development of his art. And the world has easily forgotten that from the day of Paganini, not only was the violin transformed into a new instrument, not only were its capabilities, previously undreamt of, newly revealed; but also in other branches of musical art, in orchestral music especially, a fresh field was opened up before the composer. It is scarcely too much to say that the scores of Tchaikovsky and Richard Strauss could not have been written, had Paganini never lived. We do not desire to see another Paganini, so complete a slave to his instrument, albeit its master; we do not desire to see another such life, with bodily health and moral vigour sacrificed to so absorbing a devotion to one single end. We would fain believe that Nicolo Paganini did not live in vain, that like a real artist he had and fulfilled his mission, that the evil he did died with him and that the good lives on to benefit the world."

REFERENCES

Nicolo Paganini, His Life and His Works.   By Stephen S. Stratton.
The Dictionary of Music.

JOHANN FREDERIC SCHILLER

JOHANN CASPAR SCHILLER, a barber-surgeon in the Bavarian army, being temporarily without employment, was on his way home when he chanced to stop for the night at the Golden Lion Inn at Marback, in Wurttemberg. Here he fell in love with the landlord's daughter, Dorothea, and, a few months later, married her. To them was born, on November 10, 1759, a son who was christened Johann Christoph Friedrich Schiller. Friedrich was the second child in the family. Of his five sisters, two died in infancy.

The father finally retired from the army, with the rank of captain, and became head forester for the Duke of Würtemberg, at Castle Solitude, his estate at Ludwigsburg. Here the boy Schiller spent his childhood amid very happy surroundings. With his sister he was sent to the village school, where he proved himself so apt a pupil that he was sent to the village pastor for instruction in Latin. He conceived a great admiration for the minister and resolved to become a preacher himself. Since his parents were of a very religious nature they heartily approved of his ambition.

This hope was not to be realized, for the Duke of Würtemberg, wearying of the wild and extravagant life he had been leading, turned to philanthropy and founded a school for boys, first at Solitude and, later, moved it to Stuttgart. The school was founded for the sons of his military officers, but approving of both Schiller and his father, he invited the former to enter the school. This was not altogether to the liking of the Schiller family, for it precluded any possibility of the ministry; but rather than offend the Duke, Schiller was enrolled in 1773, for six years of bondage.

The school was conducted on the rigid routine plan of a military academy. Visits to and from parents were prohibited and all letters went through the hands of the intendant. Schiller had taken up the study of law in his second year, not from choice, but because the Duke had suggested it. In 1775, a department of medicine was established and, though that was almost equally distasteful he turned to it as the lesser of two evils.

With some friends he founded a literary club which read and discussed any and all books that could be smuggled to them. Presently they were inspired to do a little writing themselves and, for the first time, dreams of literary fame began to take form in Schiller's mind. Such relics of his poetry and essays, as remain from his school days, had little promise of the power to come—but they served as a beginning. His attention being turned toward drama, he plunged into the ecstasies of producing his first play. To gain time for writing he feigned illness and worked with feverish energy on "The Robbers," his first play.

For a time Schiller dropped his literary pursuits to bend all his energies on a thesis which he hoped might secure his release from the hateful school routine a year earlier; but it was condemned as tedious and unfit for print. He worked hard whenever possible throughout the year, on "The Robbers" which was virtually finished in June, 1780. In November of the same year he submitted another thesis, which was accepted; but instead of procuring him the desired liberty from routine, with leisure to write, he was appointed doctor to a regiment stationed at Stuttgart, on a small salary. This meant that he must still wear a uniform and submit to a certain measure of routine. He was not even allowed to extend his practice among the people of the city and thereby to add a bit to his scanty pay. He was greatly disappointed, after studying for seven years, to find that he must hold such a position, offering no opportunity for development.

In the hope of making a little money, Schiller planned to publish "The Robbers." As with most beginners, he did not meet with great success; so he decided to borrow money and print the play at his own expense. Fortunately, his work had not long to depend on its own literary merit. Schwann, a bookseller in Mannheim, after reading it, was convinced that it had great dramatic merit and he took it to Baron Dalberg, manager of the Mannheim theater. Dalberg realized its value and wrote to Schiller, offering to produce it if it was revised and made more practical for the stage. The play was practically rewritten, before Dalberg was satisfied, but it was finally produced on the 12th of January, 1782, when it was very favorably accepted.

It was now harder than ever for Schiller to settle down in Stuttgart, calling upon and treating sick soldiers. Nevertheless, he had no other choice. The Duke learned of the visit to Mannheim and put Schiller under arrest for two weeks, because the visit had not been authorized by him. The Duke was incensed also, at some of the sentiments expressed in "The Robbers" and informed Schiller that he was to attend to business and write no more "comedies." Schiller then wrote a very humble letter to the Duke, in which he begged to be allowed time and liberty to continue his work. The Duke replied to the effect that Schiller would be arrested again if he did not immediately drop the subject. By this time Schiller saw the absolute impossibility of any development there, so he decided to leave Würtemberg.

He divulged his plans to only a few close friends. Frau von Wolzogen offered him her house, in Bauerbach, as a quiet refuge. He had planned to go to Mannheim and put himself under the employment of Dalberg, but Dalberg was afraid that the Duke might become informed of Schiller's whereabouts and consequently declined his employment. Then Schiller accepted the offer of shelter at Bauerbach and settled down in the little cottage placed at his disposal. He began to revise "Fiesco," said to be the weakest of Schiller's plays. Dalberg steadily refused to produce it and he finally sold it to Schwann, who published it in book form. Schiller now began to work on a tragedy, entitled "Louise Miller" and again submitted it to Dalberg, who was now in a more friendly frame of mind and urged the author to come to Mannheim and work on its revision for the stage, now known under the

title of "Cabal and Love." This was so well
received that Dalberg began to consider "Fiesco,"
which he had previously rejected; and when this
had been revised and produced, Schiller's success
as a man of letters seemed assured. Dalberg
then offered him a year's contract as dramatist
to the Mannheim theater with a fairly good
salary, and the future looked brighter. The contract provided for one entirely new play a year,
besides those already on hand. Unfortunately,
Schiller fell ill, and was unable to work for some
months, meanwhile falling badly in debt. Apparently, Dalberg did not understand Schiller's
condition, for he refused to renew the contract
and suggested that Schiller had better go back
to medicine.

Schiller had hoped to be able to start a dramatic journal; and, having lost his position with
Dalberg, he began the preparation of the first
number. He was too hopeful, however, as the
subscriptions proved entirely inadequate to publish it. A little later, a letter came from Leipzig,
from four anonymous writers, expressing their
regard and esteem for Schiller and his works.
Schiller did not answer for some time; but following his eventual reply, a correspondence developed between him and Gottfried Korner,
which soon convinced him that he ought to be

in Leipzig with these people. Already he had begun work on "Don Carlos" the first act of which fell into the hands of the Duke of Weimar, while he was visiting near Mannheim. The Duke was so pleased with it that he conferred upon Schiller the title of Weimar Councillor which, though it brought him no income, gave him an honorable status among the German people.

Schiller, believing that he was not properly appreciated in Mannheim, wrote to Korner that he was coming to Leipzig to make his acquaintance with his, as yet unknown, friends. Korner was a friend indeed, for he advanced Schiller enough money to pay his most pressing debts, and, having an interest in the publishing business, agreed to take over Schiller's proposed magazine, known as the "Thalia." Korner was about to be married and it was arranged that, after the marriage, Schiller should take up his residence in Dresden with them. This was his home for the next two years and it was a happy one. From Korner he received exactly the kind of intellectual stimulus he most needed, and from that period dates some of his finest poetry. In Mannheim he had lost most of his enthusiasm for the theater, which now began to revive, and he started working on a stage version of "Don Carlos" for the Hamburg theater. With this completed, Schiller set out on a visit to Weimar, to return no more to Dresden excepting for an occasional visit.

He remained for some time in Weimar, hoping for the return of Goethe who was then in Italy. From there he went to visit a professor at Jena, who assured him it would be easy to secure a professorship at the University if he desired it. He did not at once make up his mind in the matter, and went back to Weimar, where he met Charlotte von Lengefeld who became his wife a year later. In the spring of 1789, he was appointed professor of history at Jena, and though he had but a very small salary, he decided it justified his marriage and in February, 1790, Lotte von Lengefeld and Schiller were wed.

The year 1790 is said to have been the happiest in Schiller's life. He and his wife were perfectly happy and, though his income was small, his courage was great. Unfortunately, while spending his vacation with friends, in the winter of 1791, Schiller took a cold which developed into pneumonia. The condition was treated lightly and unsuccessfully and he returned to Jena and his work in poor health. Soon another attack occurred, this time accompanied by hemorrhages and other suspicious symptoms. For many days it seemed that he would not recover. Then he began to show evidence of a slight improvement, which proved to be extremely slow. He had consumption and for a long time complained of pain in the right side of his chest, as well as of marked shortness of breath. He was able to secure a release from his professorship through the Duke of Weimar, and in the spring he grew strong enough to begin a second installment of the "Thirty Years War," begun in 1789.

Schiller took up his abode in Rodolstadt and there, in May, he was prostrated by a relapse, which proved worse than the first attack. It was months before he was able to think of reading or writing; and he was now in serious financial straits, since his illness had been very costly. But help came unexpectedly from Denmark, where were two noblemen, his fervid admirers, hearing that he was sick and very much in need of money, sent him a gift of a thousand thalers a year for three years, during which time he was to rest and be free from anxiety. For the first time in his life, Schiller was free to form his own plans and to take his own time. At first he continued to reside in Jena, where he started a new "Thalia." When spring came he decided to try the climate of his native Suabia, and since the Duke of Würtemberg was no longer hostile, he spent almost a year with his family and friends.

In May, 1794, he returned to Jena. His health had not improved and as a physician he knew that he had but few more years to live. The knowledge seemed to stimulate him, for he felt that he still had much to do. He threw all his energy into a literary magazine, known as *Die Horen.* He invited the coöperation of all the best writers in Germany, among them Goethe, and thus began a correspondence which developed into a great friendship. Goethe accepted Schiller's invitation, for he was beginning to be weary of his life at Weimar, and said that he would not only contribute, but would serve on the editorial staff of the new journal. They met a few days later, in Jena, and though the acquaintance began with an argument, they had too great an admiration for each other's powers to disagree long, and both craved comradeship. A little later Schiller spent two weeks in Weimar as Goethe's guest, where they laid the foundation of a life-long friendship.

The *Horen* was not a success at the beginning. It was too profound for the ordinary reader. But, as time went on, it grew popular and though it only lasted for three years, its end came by mutual consent of editor and publisher and was not due to failure. In the fall of 1796, Schiller began "Wallenstein" and from that time on dramatic poetry was his chief interest. He led a quiet life, often ill and depressed, but very resolute, and finding much happiness in his own home and in the friendship of Goethe. "Wallenstein," which was cast in three parts, was put upon the Weimar stage, on January 30, 1779, under Schiller's personal direction, marking his return to drama and accounted by many as his masterpiece.

Almost immediately after the completion of "Wallenstein," Schiller planned "Mary Stuart." He first began a version of "Macbeth" for the Weimar theater; but, before he could finish it, he was prostrated with another long attack of his malady. In 1800, he went to Ettersburg, and there completed his tragedy of the Scottish queen. It was staged almost at once and has remained one of his accepted dramatic productions. "The Maid of Orleans," a romantic tragedy, based on the historical Joan of Arc, was finished in 1801. He spent several weeks that summer with Korner in Dresden, doing no writing. After trying several subjects, "The Bridge of Messina" was completed in 1803. There seems to be a wide difference of opinion as to its merits.

Schiller's last play, like his first, was inspired by the sentiment of freedom; but it was of a much milder character and indicated the writer's increased experience and wisdom. It was another illustration of its author's versatility. It was utterly different from any of his other plays. "William Tell," by far the most human, is the only one which does not end with a tragic note. Its first performance, in 1804, was most enthusiastically received, and ever since it has been one of the favorites of the German stage.

After the completion of "William Tell" Schiller began "Warbeck"; and then the story of Dmitri, the son of Ivan the Terrible. Before much work was done upon these, however, he decided to go to Berlin, where he had long been urged to come, and left for the German capital with his wife and children in the spring of 1804. He was most cordially received by the king and queen and inducements were offered him to remain there. He did not really wish to leave Weimar and his friends; so went to the Duke and told him of the offer to come to Berlin. The Duke of Weimar promptly doubled his stipend and Schiller was very willing to let it now appear impossible for him to leave.

He began working again on "Warbeck," but, in February, 1805, he was prostrated again and it was very evident that his end was near. He tried to work a little more and, on April 29, he went to the theater. The effort proved too much, and though he lingered on for a few days, his death occurred on May 9, 1805. He was buried at Weimar, in the churchyard of St. James; but, in 1826, his remains were exhumed and taken to the ducal mausoleum, where they now rest near the tomb of Goethe and of the Duke himself. He had led a secluded life and it was not, perhaps, until later years that the world fully realized that one of the Immortals had passed on into the temple of eternal fame.

REFERENCES

Life of Schiller. By Thomas Carlyle.
Life and Works of Schiller. By Calvin Thomas.

XAVIER BICHAT

MARIE FRANCOIS XAVIER BICHAT, was born November 11, 1771, at Thoirette, in the province of Bresse, now known as the department of Jura. His father, Jean Baptiste Bichat, was a physician as well as mayor of Poncin in Bugey. The father strongly desired that his son should become a physician and consequently taught him much about medicine. Although Bichat was always a brilliant child we have no record of any outstanding events in his early life. Having decided upon medicine as a career, his father sent him to Lyons, where he studied under Antoine Petit.

During his school days he was interested in mathematics and physics; consequently he began to apply the methods he had learned in those subjects to the study of the structure of the human body, anatomy. For a time he returned home to help his father; but it was not long before he went back to Lyons to further his education, particularly in mathematics and anatomy. Then came the French Revolution and with it the closing of the schools in Lyons. Very fortunately, Bichat went to Paris to study, where he found better training and broader channels into which to direct his energies. He knew no one in Paris, neither did he have an approachable manner, but he did not regard this as a hindrance. He entered the school of Desault, generally regarded as the greatest surgeon of his time. The following incident, related by one of Bichat's biographers, brought about a very happy relationship between the great teacher and his pupil. "It was an established custom in the school of Desault that certain chosen pupils should undertake to make notes, in turn, of the public lesson and should prepare an abstract. This abstract was read after the lesson of the following day; and these exercises, presided over by the associate surgeon, had the double advantage of bringing a second time before the pupils the useful precepts which they should absorb, and of compensating for the sufficiently common inattention of the masses during the first lesson. One day, when Desault had spoken for a long time on a fracture of the clavicle, and had demonstrated the utility of his bandage, applying it at the same time to a patient, the pupil whose duty it was to note these details happened to be absent. Bichat offered to take his place. The reading of his abstract caused a real sensation. The

purity of his style, the precision and clearness
of his ideas, the scrupulous exactness of his
resumé, were characteristic rather of the
professor than the pupil. He was heard with
extraordinary attention and left showered with
praise and repeated applause." As a result,
Desault took him into his home and made him
his assistant. This association was a delight,
as well as an inspiration to Bichat; but its duration was relatively short. Desault died suddenly
in 1795. Besides taking up Desault's work
where he had left it, and preparing it for the
publisher, the care of his widow and her son was
left to Bichat. In this way, he partially ac-
quitted himself of the obligation under which he
had been placed. He abandoned his own researches, in which he was deeply immersed; and
conducted to a close the fourth volume of Desault's unfinished *Journal de Chirurgie*, bringing
it up to the very highest standard by help of his
own originality and powers of expression.

At that time, anatomy was in a state of chaos,
as evidenced by the following appreciation:
"Up to that time, bristling with scholastic
minutiae, anatomy repelled too often by its
dryness the young who were destined to the
study of the healing art. We cannot even today
recall, without a sensation of pain, all those

multiple divisions, those fatiguing descriptions, that conventional and often incomprehensible language which constituted then the science of anatomy. Bichat was the first to leave the common path. He presented anatomy from a new point of view; he studied the general organization of man in the simple tissues of which the body is composed; he divided the living economy into various systems, and by accumulating facts, by bringing observation to bear on experience, he broadened the limits of science and built for himself a monument which brings him lasting renown."

Bichat entered this field with great fervor. He cast aside the old time methods and substituted actual observation and experiment. He devoted himself diligently to this work throughout the day and far into the night. His careful observation were followed by accurate descriptions of what he saw. Soon his work attracted attention and physicians and pupils began to gather around him. A demand was created for private instruction; and therefore, in 1797, his first course in anatomy was organized. This new work greatly stimulated him and he continued to plunge into various phases of his studies with dangerous fervor. He, with Corvisart, was instrumental in organizing the

Société Médicale d'Émulation. In 1800, he published his first great book on anatomy. In this
he took great strides toward wresting anatomy
from its chaotic state. He said: "Chemistry has
its simple bodies. In like manner anatomy has
its simple tissues, which by their combinations
form the organs." Again he said: "As every
tissue has everywhere a similar disposition,
since, wherever it may be, it possesses the same
structure, the same properties, etc., so it is clear
that its diseases must be everywhere the same.
Whether the serous tissue belongs to the brain
as the arachnoid, to the lungs as the pleura, to
the heart as the pericardium, to the abdominal
viscera as the peritoneum, etc., it takes on in-
flammation everywhere in the same way, everywhere dropsies occur in the same way," etc.
Then, in the same year, and following closely
upon the heels of this great book, came a greater
one, covering the results of his physiological
researches upon the living and the dead. When
he was only twenty-nine years old he had been
appointed adjunct physician to the Hotel Dieu.
This position gave him wonderful opportunities
to further his observations on the living, as well
as on the dead, body. Indeed, it is said that
during a single winter he made between 600 and
700 post-mortem examinations. All of his valu-

able experiences and observations he recorded in the manuscripts of his books. He worked with great speed and accuracy. It is said, indeed, that he would write so fast, and that his manuscripts would be so accurate, that they would not have to be re-read or corrected before publication. He believed so strongly in observation and thought the reading of books was not of much value to him. On this point he once said: "If I have gone forward so rapidly, the result has been that I have read little. Books are merely the memoranda of facts. But are such memoranda necessary in a science whose material is ever near us; where we have, so to speak, living books in the sick and the dead? Let us halt when we have arrived at the limits of the most careful and thorough observation, and let us not strive to press forward where experience cannot show us the way."

In 1801, he came forth with another book, of which Cersie said: "Pathological anatomy, which was but a collection of isolated facts, is here raised to the rank of a science. Medical genius has never at a single bound raised itself to so great a height." In the preface of this marvelous book, Bichat says: "Experiments on living animals, tests with various reagents on organized tissues, dissections, necropsies, observa-

tion of man in health and disease, these are the
sources from which I have drawn; they are those
of nature. Nor have I neglected those of the
authors, especially of those from whom the
science of the animal economy has been a science
of facts and experience." In this same book
his great vision of the future of medicine and of
the relationship between its various phases is
expressed as follows: "We are, it seems to me,
at a point where pathological anatomy must
take a new flight. It is not alone the science
of those changes which primarily or secondarily
develop gradually in the course of chronic disease;
it includes the examination of every alteration
to which our parts are subject at whatsoever
period of the disease. How petty are the reason-
ings of a multitude of physicians, great in the
eye of the public, when investigated not by the
light of their own writings, but in the cadaver!
Medicine has been for a long time excluded from
the exact sciences; it will have a right to be associated with them at least as regards the diagnosis of disease when one shall have combined
everywhere with rigorous clinical observation
the examination of the alterations suffered by
our organs. Of what value is clinical observation if one is ignorant of the seat of evil? You
might take notes at the bedside of the sick for

twenty years, from morning to night, on affec-
tions of the heart, of the lungs, of the abdominal
viscera, etc., and there will be but confusion in
the symptoms, which resting upon no certain
base, will of necessity bring before you an in-
coherent sequence of phenomena. Open a few
cadavers and that obscurity which clinical observation alone could never have dissipated will
vanish in a moment from before your eyes."

Bichat was interested not only in anatomy,
but also in the treatment and the diagnosis of
disease. It was he who conceived the idea of
dividing certain diseases of the chest formerly
grouped under one name into pleuritis, pneumonia, and bronchitis.

Bichat had worked extremely hard all his life
and now, after giving to the world such a wealth
of knowledge in so brief a period of time, he
rushed forward, with the same dangerous fervor, into the preparation of a series of volumes on
descriptive and pathological anatomy. Long
ere they were finished, his health broke. He
began to have hemorrhages from the lungs. He
had consumption. Nevertheless he remained
undaunted in his purpose, and at times, when
it was impossible for him to be very active
physically, he thought out and planned his works
for publication. He was known to return again

and again, to his work when he was not fit physically. After each illness, he plunged into his labors with the same ardour as before, hardly giving his body a fair chance to regain its former vigor and endurance, until one day, while working in the foul atmosphere of decomposing bodies, he had an attack of dizziness and on leaving his laboratory fell on the stairs, striking his head violently. This attack proved too great for his health which was badly broken from consumption. On July 22, 1802, he died in the arms of Mrs. Desault, who had served as a real mother to him since the time he entered their home as her husband's assistant.

Bichat had laid his life upon the altar of science. When he died he did not have enough money to bury him, but he left behind him that which is far greater than money. So many were his friends that upon learning of his death they rushed to the scene; took the best of care of his dead body; and all the faculty, together with 600 students, followed it to the grave in St. Catherine Cemetery. Forty-three years later, the body was exhumed and carried to Notre Dame. Thousands of people were in the funeral procession, including 4,000 members of the medical profession, as the body was carried for re-interment at Pére-La-chaise.

The famous Corvisart, who was to play so prominent a rôle in the life of Laennec and who became Napoleon's personal physician, wrote to Bonaparte as follows: "Bichat has just died at the age of 30; he has fallen upon a field of battle which, also, calls for courage, and which counts many a victim; he has broadened the science of medicine; no one at his age has done so many things and done them so well." Upon receiving this letter, Napoleon wrote to the Minister of the Interior as follows: "I beg that you will place in the Hotel Dieu a marble dedicated to the memory of Citizens Desault and Bichat which shall attest the gratitude of their contemporaries for the service which they have rendered, the one to French surgery, of which he was the restorer; the other to medicine, which he has enriched by many useful works. Bichat would have broadened the domain of this science, so important and so dear to humanity, if pitiless death had not struck him down at the age of 30."

If Bichat could have enlisted the aid of the microscope, there can be no estimate as to what greater service he would have brought his vast store of knowledge. Although he did not have that aid, the science of anatomic structure is based directly upon the facts he disclosed; and hence, he is properly called the *father of histology*. As time passes, the world's recognition of his greatness increases. Thayer has said: "His observations and methods of research are models for all time." Buckle says: "Great, however, as is the name of Cuvier, a greater still remains behind. I allude, of course, to Bichat, whose reputation is steadily advancing as our knowledge advances; who, if we compare the shortness of his life with the reach and depth of his views, must be pronounced the most profound thinker and consummate observer by whom the organization of the animal frame has yet been studied." "We may except Aristotle, but between Aristotle and Bichat I find no middle man."

REFERENCES

Biology and Its Makers. By William A. Locy.
Xavier Bichat, His Life and Labors. By R. Knox, M.D. *Lancet*, Vol. II, 1854.

RENE THEODORE LAENNEC

IN ALL medical history there is no more fascinating chapter than that concerning the discovery of the stethoscope. The fact that the discoverer of the stethoscope, Laennec, was himself a sufferer from tuberculosis and, later, died of this disease adds greatly to its interest. In the face of great suffering and handicap, he became one of the foremost physicians of all time. Laennec was born at Quimper, in Bretagne, on February 17, 1781. His father was a lawyer, although he devoted a great deal of his time to literature and particularly, to the writing of poetry. Laennec's mother died when he was but six years old, and because his father seemed too busy to care for him, he was placed in charge of a grand-uncle, a priest in the Catholic Church. At the hands of this relative he received excellent care, special attention being paid to ventilation and to hygienic conditions in general. His uncle provided him, also, with good mental training. After some five years, Laennec went to live with a paternal uncle, who was a physician and a member of the Faculty of Medicine at the University of Nantes. Here

Laennec devoted himself assiduously to his school work and although his education, like everything else in the days of the French Revolution, was seriously interrupted, his good scholarship won for him numerous prizes. Nevertheless, conscious that in certain respects his training was deficient, he went at the age of nineteen years, to Paris, where he again took up the study of Latin and pursued it until he could write and speak that language fluently. He was already well versed in English and German.

Becoming interested, through the influence of his uncle, in medicine he entered the medical school of the University of Paris. Here again he worked so diligently that he was awarded the first prize in both medicine and surgery. During his University course he became a pupil and admirer of Corvisart,—a very practical man. Corvisart had brought into common use among physicians that form of physical examination known as percussion, although it had been carefully worked out and described by Auenbrugger nearly fifty years before. Napoleon Bonaparte selected Corvisart as his personal physician. Through his association with this progressive physician and with other able associates, Laennec received an excellent training, not alone in the practice of medicine, but also in methods of scientific investigation. For several years after graduation he spent his time in the observation and care of hospital patients, and in a number of fatal cases he had the opportunity to study conditions post-mortem. He was deeply interested in the structure of the normal human body, having early become a prominent member of the Anatomical Society of France. He devoted much time to the study of deviations from the normal, resulting from diseases of various organs, and unquestionably it was his careful investigations at the post-mortem table that materially aided him in making his eventual contributions to the relief of humanity. During this early period he made a number of valuable additions to medical literature. As early as 1804, he wrote two papers upon the Life and Work of Hippocrates, the ancient Greek physician. In the same year he published a description of the membranes investing the liver. Later on, he described changes in the liver due to the use of alcohol and this condition became known as Laennec's or alcoholic cirrhosis. An excellent article upon peritonitis appeared from his pen. All of these illustrate the breadth of his interest in medicine at large.

In 1816, he was appointed physician to the Necker Hospital. Already he was growing famous in his profession, and physicians came from all parts of the civilized world to be taught of him. He is said to have been an ideal teacher, appearing before his classes with lectures and illustrative material always prepared with great care. His presentation was simple, employing the conversational method and yet his message was delivered with such great force that he always made a deep and lasting impression upon his students.

Then came that great outstanding invention, predicted more than a century before, when Walshe said: "Who knows but that one may discover the works performed in the several offices and shops of a man's body by the sounds they make and may thereby discover what instrument or organ is out of order!" Laennec devised the stethoscope and because of it his name has been immortally graven upon the walls of fame. His own description of this discovery follows: "In 1816, I was consulted by a young person who was laboring under the general symptoms of a diseased heart. In her case percussion and the application of the hand (which modern doctors call palpatation) were of little service, because of a considerable degree of stoutness. The other method, that namely of listening to the sounds within the chest by the

direct application of the ear to the chest wall,
being rendered inadmissible by the age and sex
of the patient, I happened to recollect a simple
and well known fact in acoustics and fancied it
might be turned to some use on the present
occasion. The fact I allude to is the great dis-
tinctness with which we hear the scratch of a
pin at one end of a piece of wood on applying
our ear to the other.

"Immediately on the occurrence of this idea
I rolled a quire of paper into a kind of cylinder
and applied one end of it to the region of the
heart and the other to my ear. I was not a
little surprised and pleased to find that I could
hereby perceive the action of the heart in a
manner much more clear and distinct than I
had ever been able to do by the immediate
application of the ear.

"From this moment I imagined that the circumstance might furnish means for enabling us
to ascertain the character not only of the action
of the heart, but of every species of sound produced by the motion of all the thoracic viscera,
and consequently for the exploration of the
respiration, the voice, the râles and perhaps even
the fluctuation of fluid effused in the pleura or
pericardium. With this conviction I forthwith
commenced at the Necker Hospital a series of

observations from which I have been able to deduce a set of new signs of the diseases of the chest. These are for the most part certain, simple, and prominent, and calculated, perhaps, to render the diagnosis of the diseases of the lungs, heart and pleura as decided and circumstantial as the indications furnished to the surgeons by the finger or sound in the complaints wherein these are of use."

Although the instrument Laennec invented and described was simple—and the stethoscope remained simple during his lifetime—it has since been greatly elaborated, and yet no one within the century and more that has passed since his discovery, has made more satisfactory descriptions of sounds heard from within the chest than he made. Indeed, at the time Laennec discovered the stethoscope, knowledge of diseases of the heart and lungs was in a chaotic state. He also interpreted the sounds coming to the ear from the lungs so that he was able to differentiate between various diseases. Previous to this time, *lung fever* was a common diagnosis. Because of the lack of differential knowledge, most abnormal conditions of the lungs, accompanied by fever, were then called *lung fever*. With his newly invented stethoscope, however, Laennec pointed out the difference between such diseases as pleurisy, pneumonia and bronchitis. He then described with great accuracy the sounds, heard over the lungs, resulting from the different forms and phases of tuberculosis; from pulmonary cancer and several other of the less common respiratory diseases. Laennec's interpretations of sounds coming from the heart were not entirely correct; but, nevertheless, he laid down the principles upon which accurate diagnostic signs of various abnormal heart conditions are based today.

After long and careful study of the sounds heard from within the chest, Laennec published, in 1819, a book upon the subject. So great was the demand for it that the first edition was exhausted by 1823. A second edition was demanded. Since the appearance of the first, Laennec had continued his studies with the stethoscope, so that he was able to make many valuable additions to the work. In fact, he wrote an entirely new book. So fundamental were the principles laid down in this edition and so slight are the changes in our later knowledge of the subject that it is read with great profit by physicians and students of medicine to this day.

In the preface of the work, he declares: "I may say that no one who has made himself expert with this method will after this have occasion to say, with Baglivi, 'Oh! how difficult it is to diagnose disease of the lungs.'

"For our generation is not inquisitive as to what is being accomplished by its sons. Claims of new discoveries, made by contemporaries, are likely for the most part to be met by smiles and mocking remarks. It is always easier to condemn than to test by actual experience.

"It suffices for me if I can only feel sure that this method will commend itself to a few worthy and learned men who will make it of use to many patients. I shall consider it ample, yea, more than sufficient reward for my labor, if it should prove the means by which a single human being is snatched from untimely death."

Laennec dressed very plainly and it is said that, instead of supporting beautiful carriages, as many less important physicians did, he usually hired a cab. He lived a simple, self-sacrificing life of service, always inspired by the burning desire to prolong life and to prevent suffering of others. As he said in his preface, he was sufficiently rewarded for his work if it should prove to be the means of saving one human being from untimely death. It is said that after he became famous he often refused to go to see wealthy patients, but that he never on any occasion refused his services to the poor.   He was a devout member of the Catholic Church.   Austin Flint, one of the most expert physicians in diseases of the chest that America has ever produced said: "Laennec's life affords an instance, among many others, disproving the vulgar error that the pursuits of science are unfavorable to religious faith.   He lived and died a firm believer in the truths of Christianity.   He was a truly moral and a sincerely religious man."

In writing of Laennec's death, Bayle, who lived contemporaneously with Laennec, said: "His death was that of a true Christian, supported by the hope of a better life; prepared by the constant practice of virtue, he saw his end approach with composure and resignation.   His religious principles, imbibed with his earliest knowledge, were strengthened by the convictions of his maturer reason.   He took no pains to conceal his religious sentiments when they were disadvantageous to his worldly interests, and he made no display of them when their avowal might have contributed to favor and advancement.

"He never imposed upon others.   Only two hours before his death he took the rings from his fingers and placed them upon a table.   When his wife asked why he did this, he said: 'It will not be long now before someone else would have to do this service for me, and I do not wish that they would have the trouble.' "

Writing of Laennec, Austin Flint said: "In his character were beautifully blended the finest intellectual and moral qualities of our nature. With mental powers of the highest order were combined simplicity, modesty, purity, and disinterestedness in such measure that we felt he was a man to be loved not less than admired. His zeal and industry in scientific pursuits were based on the love of truth for its own sake and a desire to be useful to his fellow-men. To these motives to exertion much of his success is to be attributed. Mere intellectual ability and acquirements do not qualify either to make or to appreciate important scientific discoveries. The mind must rise above the obstruction of self-love, jealousy and selfish aims. Hence it is that most of those who have attained to true eminence in the various paths of scientific research have been distinguished for excellencies of the heart as well as of the head. The example of Laennec is worthy of our imitation. His superior natural gifts we can only admire, but we can imitate the industry without which his genius would have been fruitless. Let us show our reverence to the memory of Laennec by endeavoring to follow humbly in his footsteps."

Throughout his life, Laennec was in somewhat delicate health. Indeed when he went to live with his grand-uncle his health had to be carefully guarded. Through the excellent care he received, however, he was able to carry on his studies successfully while in school and to preform his duties excellently after entering upon the practice of medicine. Because of his intense interest in people who were ill, his burning desire to help them and his never-ending labor in his attempts to contribute to medical knowledge in such a way as to relieve the whole human family from suffering and untimely death, he overtaxed his strength. The first break in health came in 1806, but it did not seem serious. In fact, he remained in Paris, continued a part of his work and was able soon to resume all of his duties. In 1819, his nerves failed him. Because of these symptoms he was unable to work, so he went to Kerlouanec where he spent about two years as nearly as possible free from mental work, and engaged in field and other sports in the open air. With much improved health, he returned to Paris where he resumed his customary pursuits. Only one year later, he was appointed Professor of Medicine in the College of France and his practice as well as his other duties increased so rapidly that it was not long before he again showed evidence of failing health. Within four years he had acquired a severe cough, he had lost weight, had developed a fever and was suffering from pleurisy. He had tuberculosis of the lungs and now he felt sure that his two previous attacks were manifestations of the same disease. He went back to Kerlouanec and the change brought about a temporary improvement. At that time bleeding, which had been practised by the ancients in treating many diseases, was still employed in the treatment of tuberculosis. Laennec had much blood drawn from his veins. One can scarcely imagine anything more harmful than the taking of the life-blood of which he already had too little and for which he stood in so great need. From time to time his attacks grew more severe and he became weaker and weaker. He came to the conclusion that he was suffering from "galloping" consumption. His long study of tuberculosis and his resulting written work on the subject justify one in saying that no one had lived before him whose knowledge of tuberculosis could approach his. In consequence, he was well aware of what was going on in his own case and he understood clearly, out of his own observation, that the end was not far distant. Indeed, at one time, he predicted that he could live but eight days, and although his prediction was not exactly correct he was making his last stand against the disease. During his last illness he worked on the second edition of his famous book. Unquestionably this labor took much of his strength, but he succeeded in finishing the book before he died and so greatly enriched the world's knowledge of tuberculosis.

Laennec was a firm believer in the beneficial effects of the sea-air; so he requested that his windows be kept wide open day and night; during the day, he often spent much time sitting in a chair in which he had been carried out under the trees. Upon many of the last days of his illness he insisted upon riding out in a carriage twice daily. As the end approached his hope of recovery increased, but he grew weaker and weaker, in part as a result of the treatment he received, and he died on August 13, 1826.

Thus Laennec who had fought so hard to prevent the untimely death of others fell upon his own battle-field. He knew more about the enemy he had to fight than any other living man, yet he entirely forgot himself in his strenuous efforts to save others. Through his discoveries and his interpretation of his findings, he made the detection of early tuberculosis possible. In our own day, no factor is more effective in reducing death-rate than this early diagnosis of the disease. Not only does its early recognition tend to prevent the spread of tuberculosis from one individual to another; but it also brings the patient under treatment at a time when excellent results are obtainable. Although Laennec died too soon, he had won his goal and, as the battle with tuberculosis continues, he must be reckoned among the greatest fighters of the disease who have ever lived. When the fight shall be over and man has been freed at last from sorrow, suffering and death from tuberculosis, Laennec's name will ring on down the ages as that of one of the great emancipators of men.

REFERENCES

Laennec, Martyr to Science. Makers of Modern Medicine. By James J. Walsh.

Glances at the Treatment of Tuberculosis in the Past. By Allen K. Krause. *The Journal of the Outdoor Life*, September, 1923.

LEIGH HUNT

L EIGH HUNT, the youngest of a large family, was born in the little village of Southgate in Middlesex, England, on October 19, 1784. His father, at the time of his son's birth, was tutor to Mr. Leigh nephew of the Duke of Chandos, and for him this youngest son was named. He had been born in the Barbados Islands and had gone to college in America. He was at first an attorney in Philadelphia, but he was forced to flee back to Barbados, and thence to England, because of his avowed royalistic tendences during the Revolution. There he turned to the pulpit and became a clergyman of more or less popularity. The mother was the daughter of a Philadelphia merchant. During early childhood Leigh would hardly recover from one illness before he was seized with another. For this reason the boy was over-delicately bred and, though the family was too poor for luxury, he was pampered and shielded at every turn, with the result that he was more than timid and far too easily frightened.

He entered Christ Hospital for his first schooling and for a time the sight of boys fighting and the fear of corporal chastisement on his own part kept him in a continual state of terror. However, though not of a disposition to give offense nor quick to take it, he became known as a romantic enthusiast and his daring in behalf of a friend or a good cause was irrepressible. In short, he could not be angered on his own account, but in support of others all dread of pain vanished and he fought with the courage for which his family was noted. He suffered much punishment for refusing to be a "fag" for anyone, but his moral courage sustained him to the end and he came through every ordeal in triumph.

At thirteen he was writing verses. His first effort was in honor of the Duke of York's "Victory at Dunkirk," a victory which turned out to be a defeat in the end, and to the author's great mortification. He spent most of his time outside of school hours, reading books.

Christ Hospital contributed to a cheerful, well-trained boyhood. Punishments were severe, sometimes, but nothing was prohibited that would not have been forbidden in a good home. Friendships formed there made the memory of the school ever dear to its students. Leigh spent the long holiday of three weeks in the country at Merton, in Surrey, with an aunt who had just come from Barbados.

At fifteen, Hunt left school; and for some time afterwards did nothing but visit school fellows, haunt the book stalls, and write verses. His father collected the verses and published them, in 1802, under the title of "Juvenilia" and Hunt says of it: "I was as proud, perhaps, of the book at that time as I am ashamed of it now." The book was so successful that unfortunately Hunt thought he had attained an end; when, in reality, it was scarcely beginning, for the poems were all imitations of greater poems, and Hunt had no style or originality of his own.

From poetry, Mr. Hunt turned to essays and later to play-writing. In this line he did not meet with the public success that his volume of poetry had achieved, but in reality his essays were far better than the poems. In 1805, John Hunt, an older brother, set up a paper called *The News*, and this offered an opportunity for Leigh to escape from the law office of his brother Stephan, in order to write the theatrical reviews for the paper. The policy of all newspapers up to this time was to give favorable notices of a new play regardless of its actual merit. *The News* decided that independence in theatrical criticism would be a novelty. At first no one believed in the sincerity of the attempt, but the paper adhered to its principle and, in a short time, Mr. Hunt though but twenty years of age was acclaimed as the foremost dramatic critic of the day.

Unfortunately, the career which promised so much received a check in the form of illness, and because Mr. Hunt persistently refused to seek the advice of a physician, for fear of having worse things foretold him, he suffered for nearly six years, trying one cure after another, in the hope of finding the right one. *He had tuberculosis!*

About 1810, the *Examiner*, the paper then edited by Mr. Hunt and his brother, began to show too strong Whig tendencies. When an article appeared denouncing the sudden change of the Prince Regent policies the proprietors were sentenced to two years imprisonment and a fine of five hundred pounds each. In spite of the possible disaster to Leigh Hunt's health from prison confinement, both he and his brother preferred to submit to a prison sentence than to accept certain bribes which were offered if they would desist in their attacks on the royal personage.

They were sentenced to imprisonment in separate jails, a disappointment to them; but surely no one ever experienced a pleasanter two years in prison than did Leigh Hunt. He entered the place on February 3, 1813, and in a month's time, by order of his physician was transferred to a ward in the infirmary, not so much because of illness as that he might enjoy as pleasant apartments as possible. He had two rooms, furnished to suit his own taste. He had his private garden where he raised choice flowers and fruit and where he sat most of the day. His family was permitted to live with him and friends called every day. In short he had every privilege of his own home, save that of liberty; and this was again returned to him on February 3, 1815. However, his regained liberty was curtailed by illness, for he was confined to his home.

In the spring of 1816, Hunt again took up his residence at Hampstead for the sake of the air; and there he finished and published the "Story of Rimini," the greater part of which had been written in prison. It was at this period that Hunt was most intimate with the three great poets of his time, Byron, Keats and Shelley. Keats, also suffering from tuberculosis, was taken ill one night almost upon the doorstep of Mr. Hunt's home, and he cared for Keats personally until he was able to be moved.

Shelley, when a youth, was sent to Hunt for counsel regarding one of his manuscripts, and the friendship between them had grown through correspondence while Hunt was in prison. When the *Examiner* was forced to close down because of declining fortunes due to the change of politics throughout Europe, it was Shelley, himself suffering from tuberculosis, who came to the rescue and urged the Hunts to come and join him in Italy. Both Mr. and Mrs. Hunt had delicate health and a change for the better in their fortunes, as well as their health, was sought in the milder climate. Mr. Hunt had never learned the value of money, a misfortune, since he had a large family to support and rainy days were numerous.

The year 1821 is memorable in shipping annals for one of the worst storms ever known on the northwest coast of Europe. The Hunts encountered its fury, for they set sail for Italy in November of that year. They managed to land at Plymouth, where Mrs. Hunt was so ill, after the fright of the voyage, that they were not able to journey toward Italy until late in the spring. This voyage was as pleasant as the winter one had been disagreeable, and the end of June found the Hunts at Leghorn with Lord Byron.

Shelley joined them there a few days later and took them to Pisa, where he also invited Keats to come for his health. The Hunts were to settle at Pisa. Shelley stayed a day or two and then started to return to Lerici for the remainder of the season. On this return voyage Shelley's boat was caught in a storm and he was drowned. His death was a terrible blow to Hunt and it was long before he recovered from the shock.

After three months at Pisa, the Hunts moved to Genoa where the projected periodical was set up. The magazine had moderate success and provided the Hunts with a livelihood although Lord Byron had anticipated greater success. In 1823, the Hunts left Genoa and moved to Florence, where they lived until September 1825, when Mr. Hunt was called back to England by the precarious fortunes of the *Examiner*. Having just published another book, written in Italy, the Hunts had the necessary funds for the journey home, which was made by easy stages in a traveling coach, since a second sea voyage was deemed too precarious.

On returning to England they lived a while at Highgate. Hunt published the *Companion*, but it failed. He attempted to start various periodicals later, but they never prospered beyond a certain circle of friendly readers. Hunt grew weaker, for his old illness had returned. Had not old friends cared for his family they would have actually suffered, for Hunt grew poorer as well as weaker. His collected verses were published by subscription in 1833 which helped his financial situation greatly. He received an invitation to write for an evening paper called the *True Sun*, but he was so weak that daily he had to be carried to his office in a coach, and very little of his writing actually found its way into the columns of the paper.

The Hunts were now settled in Chelsea, where they remained for seven years. Here Hunt contributed several articles to various papers, wrote the larger part of a book and three plays which were not published, and once more set up a paper known as *The London Journal.* His plays, which were at first rejected, scored unqualified success at Covent Garden.

He lost both his wife and his beloved youngest son, in the last years of his life, and he did not long survive them. His health continued to decline and he died on August 28, 1859. He was buried in Kensal Green Cemetery.

The secret of Hunt's success consists less in superiority of genius than of taste. His virtues were charming rather than imposing or brilliant— he had no vices but many foibles. The notoriety of some incidents in his life has deprived him of much of the honor due him for his fortitude under the severest of calamities, his unremitting literary industry under the most discouraging circumstances and his uncompromising independence as a journalist and author. He possessed every qualification of a translator and as an appreciative critic, whether literary or dramatic, he has hardly been excelled.

REFERENCES

The Autobiography of Leigh Hunt.
Leigh Hunt's Business Ability. Stories of Authors. By Edwin Watts Chubb.
Encyclopaedia Brittanica.

JOHN KEATS

THOUGH the son of an ostler in a livery stable and born in that same stable, on October 29, 1795, it was the fate of John Keats to die an Immortal at the age of twenty-five. He was the eldest son of Thomas Keats, head ostler at the Swan-and-Hoop, Finsbury Pavement, London, who married his employer's daughter and later became manager of the same establishment. Though poor, his parents had ambitions for their son and sent him to a good school at Enfield, conducted by the Rev. John Clarke. Here he became a leader through his good nature and love of battle. For those to whom the name of Keats calls to mind the delicate young man he later became, it is hard to realize the boy Keats as a youth naturally excelling in all forms of active exercise with a penchant for fighting. At the time, Keats was not attached to books, and because of his extraordinary vivacity one might easily have imagined him attaining greatness in a military capacity, rather than in literature. Indeed, as he was "born just after the Terror, his youth was exactly contemporaneous with the public career of Napoleon."

It was during these school days, when he manifested little or no interest in books, that the following occurred. "The Schoolroom: An usher is boxing the ears of his brother Tom; poor frail Tom. Little John rushes up, squares off with his fists, his eyes flashing vengeance, and drives in to the rescue."

About the age of fourteen, however, he suddenly bent all his forces to the study of books, took one prize in literature after another and, of his own free will, began to translate the *Aeneid*. From that time on, Greek mythology was his long study and deep delight; and it might be said that he became Greek in spirit, so deeply did he feel the beauty and thought of the Greek writers, even though he could know it only through translations.

In sharp contrast with the earlier school picture are the two following: "The Dining Hall: The clatter and hungry eagerness of seventy boys at the long tables. Keats has a book on his lap. He reaches out unconsciously toward the trencher, munches his ration of bread, while his eyes are intent on the pages of Bishop Burnet's 'History of My Own Time.'

"The Dormitory: It is night. The faint light from the sky reveals the row of beds and the sleeping schoolboys. One is still awake, listen-

ing with quiet rapture to the music of a pianoforte. The master's son is playing in a room
below. That same music, years after, was heard
again in an old castle on St. Agnes' Eve, 'yearning
like a god in pain.' "

The elder Keats was a man of stamina and
reticence. Unfortunately he was killed by a
fall from a horse while still in the prime of life.

In 1810, John's mother passed away, after a
long and tender nursing, in which he would suffer
no one to do anything for her except himself.
His grief at her death was very deep and real,
and for a long time he chose to hide himself
away from family and friends. His mother is
said to have been a very ordinary woman; one
whose character was conspicuous for feminine
frailties; one who was prodigal, pleasure-lov-
ing, passionate, a creature of the senses. In
spite of all this, she apparently manifested great
interest in the welfare of her four children. After
her death, the estate, consisting of eight thousand pounds, was placed in control of a guardian,
who decided that John had had enough of schooling and apprenticed him to a surgeon—a Mr.
Hammond of Edmonton. While with Mr. Hammond, Keats work consisted chiefly of holding
the horse, helping to bleed patients, and carrying
and working with drugs, in addition to reading

medicine. Thus, from observation and reading, he became quite well informed. His apprenticeship with Hammond ended in a quarrel, and in 1814 Keats went to London. There he continued to study in the hospital schools and in July, 1815, he received an appointment as dresser at Guy's Hospital. He had kept careful notes of the medical lectures and continued to study drugs and anatomy and was now a full-fledged practitioner of medicine. In that period surgery could not have been very attractive, for those were the days before anesthetics. The patient for operation was tightly strapped to a table and the surgical procedures were carried out with nothing to dull the pain except a lead bullet to clinch in his teeth. He could not writhe in pain for he was bound down. He could only groan. Those were the days, too, before antiseptics and asepsis. Surgical wounds very frequently became infected, discharged large quantities of pus and often resulted in the death of the patients. Then those were the days before artery forceps or other satisfactory devices were in use for controlling hemorrhage, when an artery was cut in certain regions of the body. It was the cutting of the temporal artery of a patient that caused Keats, in the spring of 1817, to lay down the knife and never again to take it up. During his short career as a practitioner of medicine he had shown both knowledge and skill, but the poet's mind was constantly and fast gaining ascendancy over the surgeon's hand.

The following anecdote, told by Stephens, a room-mate, shows the undercurrent in Keats rising to the surface: "One evening the two were sitting in their room, Stephens at his medical book, Keats idling, dreaming. From the candle-maker's shop below came intermittently the noise of a customer. Suddenly Keats spoke in the twilight:

" ' "A thing of beauty is a constant joy." What do you think of that, Stephens?'

" 'It has the true ring, but it is wanting in some way.'

"An interval of silence.

" ' "A thing of beauty is a joy forever." What do you think of that?'

"A moment of suspense and a prophetic judgment.

" 'That it will *live* forever.' "

Before he had given up surgery Keats was forming friendships with many young men of literary bent—George Mathew, Reynolds, Joseph Severn, Leigh Hunt and Shelley. In the same spring of 1817, that he gave up his surgical work, Keats brought forth his first volume of poems.

The book was not successful, for in the splendor of Scott and Bryon, the neophyte was lost. Published in March, sales of the volume had ceased by April. Keats went to the Isle of Wight, there planning to indulge himself in an orgy of poetry. He wrote to a friend: "I find I cannot do without poetry—without eternal poetry, half the day will not do—the whole of it. I had become all in a tremble from not having written anything of late." He wandered from the Isle of Wight to Margate and Canterbury, and finally settled, with his two brothers, in cheap lodgings at Hampstead, where he worked at "Endymion" and in the winter, for a few weeks, wrote dramatic criticisms for the *Champion*. His interest in society increased, but he cared more for informal gatherings in friendly studies, than for fashionable parties. In conversation, Keats did not shine; he preferred to sit apart and listen, or occasionally to chant verses to his delighted friends. Keats lived in a world apart from men and political affairs, content to write what was in his own heart, or to reflect some splendor of the natural world as he saw it or dreamed it to be.

In the winter of 1818, he saw much of Hunt and Shelley, and in the spring appeared his first great work, "Endymion." But at this very time, Keats had barely three years of life before him. That summer he went on a walking trip through Scotland with his friend, Charles Brown; a fatal tour, for the exposure and hardship broke his health.

Keats' mother and his brother Tom had died of consumption. During the last long illness of his mother, he was with her and cared for her almost constantly. Indeed his love for her was a big factor in his life, and her death, in 1810, was a terrible blow to him. He was a mere boy of fourteen years then, but he was strong and robust. In those days consumption was looked upon as an inherited disease and too often its contagious nature was overlooked. Think of the long and intimate contact exposure he had with his mother, in all probability the chief cause of his break in health only eight years after her death. With his medical knowledge, Keats believed his case to be hopeless, for tuberculosis was usually considered fatal in those days; and to this tragedy was added yet another—his meeting with and his hopeless love for Fanny Brawne, hopeless because of his ill health and his extreme poverty.

But despite all this, his genius continued to flame, and "The Eve of St. Agnes," "The Eve of St. Mark," and most famous of all, perhaps, his "Ode on a Grecian Urn" following in rapid succession. The latter is said to be one of the most perfect poems in the English language, and in its last two lines one finds the belief on which Keats built his life.

> Beauty is truth,—truth beauty,—that is all
> Ye know on earth, and all ye need to know.

On February 3, 1820, Keats was taken seriously ill. Hancock describes the apparent beginning of this relapse as follows: "It was one of those days of thaw and treacherous weather. Keats left his home in Hampstead without his overcoat. He rode to London on the outside of the stage-coach. Late that night he came home, flushed and fevered. Brown, with whom he was living, at Wentworth Place, advised him to go to bed at once. When he entered the bedroom a little later with medicine Keats was coughing and, spitting into the sheets, 'That is blood from my mouth,' he said. 'Bring me the candle, Brown, and let me see that blood.' In the flickering light he examined the spots on the sheet. He was a graduate in medicine. 'I know that blood,' he announced. 'It is arterial blood. I cannot be deceived in that color. That drop of blood is my death warrant. I must die.'" The instant reaction of a man's mind in a crisis which takes him unawares is one of the best tests of character. Brown, who held the candle, said that Keats looked up into his face "with a *calmness* that he could never forget."

Our views of the significance of hemorrhage have changed since 1820. Keats considered hemorrhage his death warrant. Today, we know that hemorrhage may be the first manifestation of tuberculosis and that many who have hemorrhages make complete recoveries.

After this first hemorrhage, Keats was placed on a sofa bed in the parlor, probably because he was too weak to be up; and also because from the parlor window he could observe the birds, the flowers, and some of the outside activities. Now he gained strength, but unfortunately it was not known that a cure might be effected through prolonged rest. On the contrary, it was believed that exercise should be practiced just as soon as the physical strength would permit it. Indeed, Keats took long walks when he was able to, and later changed his place of abode to Kentish Town. This all proved too much for him, for on the twenty-second of June he again began having pulmonary hemorrhages. Keats, helpless and sick, was taken into his home by Leigh Hunt who also suffered from the same disease—tuberculosis.

With the relapse of the disease, Keats became greatly discouraged and the discouragement, together with the poisons from the disease constantly being thrown into his system, definitely affected the stability of his nervous system. At times he became quite a different person. In writing to Miss Brawne he said: "I wish you could infuse a little confidence of human nature into my heart. I cannot muster any—the world is too brutal for me. I am glad there is such a thing as the grave; I am sure I shall never have any rest till I get there. I wish I were either in your arms full of faith, or that a Thunderbolt would strike me."

A little later, Keats became very indignant because a letter from Miss Brawne was delayed two days, through the negligence of a servant. He left the home of Leigh Hunt and was taken into the home of Mrs. Brawne. Although, on account of his health Keats suggested that Miss Brawne be released from her engagement, she refused to consider his suggestion and did all in her power to help her mother try to make him comfortable. This was a difficult task because of the change which had come over his mental status, and because of his declining physical condition, "the only color visible was the hectic flush on his cheeks." Even "the presence of a stranger gave him a choking sensation."

In those days, physicians believed strongly in change of climate, just as they had for more than 1600 years, since Galen sent some of his patients to Stabiae, a hill about three miles from the Bay of Naples. Here he believed they improved from consumption more rapidly than in other places. Keats' physician decided to send him to Rome, Italy, where a Dr. Clark was to be his physician. Keats thought he would never return, yet he agreed to go; and Joseph Severn arranged to accompany him. His anguish at leaving Fanny Brawne was well-nigh unbearable. He wrote to a friend: "I can bear to die, but I cannot bear to leave her. I have coals of fire in my breast. It surprises me that the human heart is capable of containing and bearing so much misery." Sailing from London, on the eighteenth of September, their boat was delayed many days because of contrary winds. When the passengers went ashore off the coast of Dorsetshire, because of the unfavorable winds, Keats wrote his last verse as follows:

> Bright star, would I were stedfast as thou art!
>   Not in lone splendor hung aloft the night,
> And watching, with eternal lids apart,
>   Like nature's patient, sleepless Eremite,
> The moving waters at their priest-like task
>   Of pure ablution round earth's human shores,
> Or gazing on the new soft-fallen mask
>   Of snow upon the mountains and the moors:

No—yet still stedfast, still unchangeable,
  Pillow'd upon my fair love's ripening breast,
To feel forever its soft-fall and swell,
  Awake forever in a sweet unrest,
Still, still to hear her tender-taken breath
And so live ever—or else swoon to death.

After the delay in the English Channel, the boat encountered a hard storm in the Bay of Biscay which lasted three days. Later it was held up and searched by a Portuguese man-of-war. Finally, upon arrival at Naples the boat was quarantined. While in Naples, Keats wrote Brown, who was with him at the time of his first hemorrhage, "I will endeavor to bear my miseries patiently. I can bear to die. I cannot bear to leave her. Oh, God! God! God! My dear Brown, for my sake, be her advocate forever."

From Naples to Rome the trip was made in a slowly moving carriage. Upon their arrival in Rome, Dr. Clark told Keats that he had only a slight affection of the lungs. Before criticising Dr. Clark too severely, the reader must remember that he did not have such modern aids as the x-ray at his disposal for determining the extent of disease. He did not even have a stethoscope, as Laennec, himself suffering from tuberculosis, did not present the possibilities of the stethoscope to the world until the next year.

It is doubtful whether anyone, under the same conditions, would have done better than Dr. Clark.

In a short time, Keats seemed to improve, just as nearly every tuberculosis patient does for a short time after a change of surroundings or climate. With this improvement, Dr. Clark prescribed short rides on horseback. At that time horseback riding was believed to be a very valuable form of treatment. Indeed it had been so regarded for about two hundred years or since the time when Sydenham so strongly advocated it. Then with this apparent improvement in health, Keats took walks out-of-doors. Indeed his last walks on earth were along the grand promenade which Napoleon had so recently constructed. At that time, walking was believed to be valuable for every patient and here again we must not criticise Dr. Clark, for he prescribed the treatment which was held to be best at that time. Nevertheless, it all proved too much for Keats, and, indeed, his improvement was only temporary. Toward the close of November he managed to do his last writing to his friend Brown, when he said: "Write to George as soon as you see this, and tell him how I am as far as you are able to guess; and also a note to my sister, who walks about my imagination like a ghost. She is so like poor Tom. I can scarcely bid you good-bye, even in a letter. *I always made an awkward bow.* God Bless you."

Somewhat before the middle of December, his health became very much worse. Dr. Clark called to see him several times every day. He was having severe hemorrhages and high fever. The next month he rallied a little and was able to take a walk, all of which Hancock has likened to "the flutter of the lamp before the darkness," for soon he suffered another attack of hemorrhages. It was during these last days, when Keats believed that he had not achieved success; that he was leaving only a few worthless fragments, that he said, as he had said months before; "If I should die, I have left no immortal work behind me, nothing to make my friends proud of my memory, but I have loved the principle of beauty in all things, and if I had had time, I would have made myself remembered." Then he prepared the following epitaph: "Here lies one whose name was writ in water,—" He requested that his name be entirely omitted from his tomb. Then he requested that, after his death, a letter from Miss Brawne that had not been opened should be wrapped in the winding sheet about his heart.

Throughout these months in Italy, Joseph

Severn was Keats' constant companion. He nursed him day and night alone; in fact, Severn did not sleep at all for the last nine days of Keats' life. What a friend! On the twenty-third of February, 1821, Keats "gradually sank into death, so quiet that I still thought he slept," wrote Severn. The post-mortem examination showed that the lungs were so badly destroyed that the physician could not understand how he lived through the last few weeks. He was buried, as Severn and Shelley were afterwards, in the Protestant Cemetery in Rome.

What a pity! Keats suffered from chronic pulmonary tuberculosis, the form now most amenable to treatment. Here, again, the blame must rest upon those who threw the world into the dark ages and who brought about the period when authority was declared the source of knowledge, even to the extent that it resulted in the complete eclipse of reason. That was the time when one who attempted to make progress in the treatment of disease did so at the risk of his very life. Had the knowledge of tuberculosis continued to increase, as it did immediately before and after the birth of Christ, perhaps Keats' life and years of service could have been greatly extended. Some say that he had already run his course, as far as literary production was

concerned; but many are inclined to believe that
had he been permitted to carry on he would have
become a close rival to Shakespeare. Be that
as it may, only a genius could accomplish all
that Keats did during so short a lifetime.

As in so many great lives, true appreciation
of his worth was not voiced until long after he
had passed. Indeed, there was much bitter
criticism of his work for sometime before and
for sometime after his death. This is especially
likely to happen to those who die young. Too
often so little credit is given to the works of
young men and young women that they become
discouraged and do not press on to the great
achievements of which they are capable. One
is reminded of the saying of long ago, "Your
young men shall see visions, and your old men
shall dream dreams." The visions of the young
should be encouraged. Consider the great accomplishments achieved by famous men and
women of the past before their thirty-fifth year
of life. Think of Keats dying at twenty-five,
a subject of severe criticism. See, as time passed
and his works were collected and analyzed, the
attitude toward him changing completely. During his lifetime his works were appreciated and
respected by but a few friends. Eight years
after his death, his poems were reprinted with a

memoir, in Paris; nineteen years after his going, a collected edition of his works was issued. A little later, a book entitled "The Life and Letters of John Keats" was published by Houghton. Then we find Keats included in "The Lives of the Illustrious," and, in 1857, duly recognized in the "Encyclopedia Britannica." Probably no greater tribute was ever paid to him than that penned by John Ruskin: "I have come to that pass of admiration for him now that I dare not read him, so discontented he makes me with my own work." Swift has expressed the general thought beautifully in his lines:

> How strange a paradox is time,
> That men who lived and died without a name
> Are the chief heroes in the sacred lists of fame.

Despite the three great misfortunes of poverty, ill-health and his hopeless love for Fanny Brawne, Keats rarely complained. His beautiful and indomitable spirit lives in all his poems. Handicapped by tuberculosis he made contributions to the world's literature which, nearly a century after his death, justify the words: "He came mysteriously out of the great deep. And, when he departed, after his brief sojourn on earth, the great deep received him again. Yet his figure abides among the imperishable memories.

He stands apart, lonely, invested with a mythical radiance, revealing unto mortals a portion of the eternal loveliness behind the veil."

REFERENCES

The Life and Letters of John Keats. By Sidney Colvin.
The Life of John Keats. By William Michael Rossetti.
Letters to Fanny Brawne.
John Keats: A Literary Biography. By Albert Elmer Hancock.
The School-days of John Keats. Stories of Authors. By Edwin Watts Chubb.
John Keats. By Amy Lowell.

ELIZABETH BARRETT BROWNING

ELIZABETH BARRETT was born on March 4, 1809, in London, the daughter of Edward Moulton-Barrett, a wealthy West Indian merchant and landowner, and Mary Clarke. The Barretts then moved to Hope End, Herefordshire, where numerous children were born. Elizabeth was her father's favorite child; on her he lavished all his affection and, very proud of her brilliant mind, he spared no pains to cultivate her intelligence. He, himself, taught her Greek and Latin in which she showed great aptitude. At nine she began to dream of being a poet and to write odes and epics after the classical examples she had been studying.

Surrounded by a happy group of children; companioned by a beloved brother, Edward, a year younger than herself, encouraged in her pursuits by a proud and indulgent father; supplied by all that wealth could procure—it is not hard to imagine that Elizabeth Barrett's childhood was a happy one. She was devoted to her books and loved riding and driving. Trying one day to saddle her pony alone, she fell and injured her spine which made her an invalid for many years. She developed a cough at this time, which persisted for ten or twelve years.

Her impaired health increased her passion for reading. She had her Greek books bound to resemble novels so that her physician would not learn about her studies and forbid them. In 1825, she contributed verses to the literary publications of the day. Her ambition prompted her to write and collect a volume of poetry, which she published anonymously in 1826. Her mother died in October, 1828, leaving Elizabeth, although an invalid, the chief consoler of her father and the guide of her seven brothers and sisters. Almost coincidently, her father lost much of his income, which he had derived from slave labor; the educated conscience of the English people demanding, by this time, the abolition of slavery. So Hope End had to be sold and the family moved to Sidmouth.

Not much is known of the home life during this period save that, in 1833, Elizabeth published a second volume of poetry which took its title from her translation in the same volume of "Prometheus Bound." After two years residence in Devonshire, the Barretts moved to London where Mr. Barrett purchased a house.

But here Elizabeth's delicate health gave way entirely, and she was confined to her couch almost continuously. The decline of health was believed to be due to the change from the pine country air and the sea breezes to the atmosphere of the city. The scientific understanding of the effects of air upon the body either in health or disease had not been proved at that time so that many opinions were held. Now that Elizabeth was compelled to be entirely inactive, she devoted herself more and more to her poetry, and published much of her work in current periodicals. Thanks to the efforts of a distant relative, John Kenyon, her poems were accepted and won the notice of an ever increasing circle of readers. But, even as her praises began to be sung, far and wide, she was suffering from what appeared to be a mortal illness. Her lungs were affected and her life seemed about to flicker out. Only her mind appeared to live, her body was almost helpless.

Towards the autumn of 1838, her condition grew very critical and her physician advised her removal to a warmer climate than London. A long journey was, of course, hazardous for her, but they succeeded in getting her safely as far as Torquay, where she was settled in comfortable apartments with her beloved brother, Edward, as her guardian. At first the mild breezes appeared to do her much good and she was able to write a little; but all the kind care of her loved ones failed of her substantial restoration to health and strength. Her studies and her poetry were pursued fitfully, during longer or shorter periods as her health would permit.

The long winter passed and with the summer the invalid seemed to be a little better. July came, and one Saturday her brother Edward arranged to go for a sail with a party of friends. They were to be gone but a few hours; but Saturday passed and the boat did not return. Mr. Barrett was not at the time with his daughter, and she had to endure the agony of suspense alone. Sunday came, and still no boat and now terrifying rumors began to creep back to the anxious ones at Torquay. Three days later on the 18th the body of one of the members of the party was picked up far down the coast. The acceptance of their fate was then unavoidable. It was not until the 4th of August that the body of Edward Barrett was discovered.

For months, Elizabeth Barrett hovered between life and death; but finally, towards the end of November, her distracted family and friends began to entertain hope for her recovery. Her one desire was to get away from all the painful memories that Torquay recalled, for the sound of the sea seemed to her the moan of a drowning man. Her return to London was not attempted until August, 1841, when the journey was made by stages of twenty-five miles a day. She stood it well, but was, of course, still a complete invalid. Happy to be home again and able once more to see her intimate friends, her health and energies appeared to revive. She wrote continually, and read and studied unceasingly. Without these interests it is doubtful if she would have lived, but in February she was able to walk from her bed to her sofa—an amazing feat for her. Her improvement was very slow, but it was sure and that was her chief concern.

Her correspondence with friends furnishes almost our only knowledge of this period, but she still wrote continuously. By February, 1843, she had prepared another volume of poems, but was at first unable to find a publisher. Not until 1844, did the book appear and by that time the collection had grown to well filled volumes. With the advent of these, fame was indeed assured for Elizabeth Barrett, and not only in England but in America.

The summer of 1846 found Miss Barrett still more or less confined to her sofa, though much improved in health. And then the most momen-

tous event of her life was at hand. Among the
few living poets, of whom she was wont to speak
with great admiration, was Robert Browning.
They had begun a correspondence, but it was
not until a comparatively short time before their
marriage that they met. How friendship ripened
into love; how each found an ideal in the other,
is one of the sweetest romances the world has
ever known. Elizabeth Barrett's exquisite "Son-
nets from the Portuguese" tell us a little of how
great was the love that inspired them. Already
in her thirty-eighth year and a confirmed invalid, it seemed that Love had passed her by,
but now it had come all unaware. The only
cloud over all her happiness was the persistent
and lasting opposition of Mr. Barrett to the
marriage of his daughter.

Mr. Barrett had extracted from all of his daughters a promise not to marry. Elizabeth had
been her father's idol; he had lavished on her
all that money or love could give. Although her
sisters knew of her correspondence the actual
marriage was withheld until her departure for
Italy, a week later, so that the wrath of her
father might not be heaped upon her sisters.
Letters which she wrote to him from Italy,
after her marriage, remained unopened; and he
even refused to see her when she came back to
England after four years of absence.

On September 12, 1846, Elizabeth Barrett and Robert Browning were married. After a week or so spent in Paris, they journeyed on by easy stages to Pisa. Mrs. Browning arrived in Pisa, not only improved in health, but fairly transformed.

They spent the winter in Pisa, where Mrs. Browning continued to improve in health and strength under the healing rays of Italy's sunshine. For some time before, and for a long time afterward, Mrs. Browning did not publish anything of importance, but neither her brain nor her pen was idle. Toward spring, Pisa grew unsuitable as a residence and the Brownings moved to Florence, and eventually settled in a romantic old palace, known as Casa Guidi, where, with some short intervals, Mrs. Browning spent the remainder of her life. She kept up her correspondence with friends in England, but rarely received any English people in her home; her usual visitors being Americans and Italians. She became, like her husband, well versed in Italian literature and lore, as well as in the political needs and social wrongs of the people. With all the strength of her remarkable character, she adopted and fought for the cause of Italy.

Thus in quiet happiness, shut in from the outer world, Robert and Elizabeth Browning dwelt in their pleasant Italian home, writing their immortal poems and content with each other's society. A further happiness was the birth of their only child, Robert Barrett Browning. The boy was startlingly like his mother, with her beautiful hair and eyes.

When the child was a little over a year old, the Brownings returned to England for the summer, and Mrs. Browning proved a revelation to all her friends who had known her only as an invalid. They made two other trips to England in succeeding years, but Florence was still their home. Here Mrs. Browning produced "Casa Guidi Windows" in 1851, and "Aurora Leigh," in 1856, referred to in those days as the finest poem ever written by a woman.

During the uprising of the Italians, in 1859, Mrs. Browning's pen and brain worked hard for the cause she had so much at heart. When the maddening treaty of peace came, just before the cause was so nearly won, Mrs. Browning was sick at heart and ill in body. She went with her husband to Siena to spend the autumn and thence to Rome, where she seemed to be again restored.

They returned to Florence and, during the year 1860, she continued to pour forth impassioned poems on behalf of Italy. In the fall of 1860 she caught a severe cold, which reactivated her lung disease and the Brownings again resorted to Rome for the winter, where the balmy air appeared to revive her once more. In May they returned to Florence and Casi Guidi, and, although she found the journey fatiguing, her friends considered that Mrs. Browning had never looked better.

She had not been in Florence more than a week before she caught another severe cold; and though some anxiety was felt, no idea of danger was entertained until the fourth night. The next day she appeared to be better again, and the worst seemed to be over. She saw an old friend or two and talked with much of her old enthusiasm. She said good-night to her little son, and only her husband watched with her on that last night. She did not suffer and did not seem conscious of approaching death, but just at dawn she begged her husband to take her in his arms, and there she died on the morning of June 29, 1861.

She was buried in the little Protestant cemetery, outside the city walls of Florence, where her grave is marked by a stately marble cenotaph, and on her home the municipality of Florence has placed a white marble slab commemorating her efforts in the cause of Italy.

Her life is a splendid example of what may

be accomplished, in spite of disease. An injury in childhood led to the development of tuberculosis which thereafter caused her great suffering and several times threatened even death; yet she pressed on and on in the face of the great handicaps of sorrow and family alienation, and eventually to a rare marriage, to a happy home, to motherhood and to the place her work won for her among the great writers of the world.

REFERENCES

Elizabeth Barrett Browning. Famous Woman Series. By John H. Ingram.
The Marriage of the Brownings. Stories of Authors. By Edwin Watts Chubb.

ST. FRANCIS OF ASSISI

IN THE ancient city of Assisi, Italy, Francesco, or Francis, was born in the year 1182. His father was a merchant and belonged to an ancient family of weavers from Lucca, while his mother came from a noble family by the name of Pica. On September 26, 1182, the baby was baptised Giovanni Bernardone. His father was in France at the time of the birth of the baby, and upon his return immediately changed the name to Francesco, or Francis.

Francis learned to speak French, though not fluently, and also studied Latin with the priests of a near-by church. This was the extent of his formal education. According to the custom in those days, Francis as the eldest son, entered the shop at an early age to assist his father. He was skillful in business, but was also very extravagant. His parents were wealthy and granted him money whenever he asked for it.

As the richest young man of the place he soon became a leader of the so-called "wild set." He entertained lavishy and all he earned was spent for pleasure. The Austere Friar Minor, from Celano, tells us the sins of these wild young

men—"they joked, were witty, said foolish
things, and wore soft, effeminate clothes."

Francis was never a strong or healthy boy.
Throughout his childhood he suffered with one
fever after another. Between 1204 and 1209 he
had many attacks of acute illness. In 1203,
during a feud he was taken prisoner and confined
in prison for almost a year, from which he
suffered severely, nearly losing his life.

However with returning health came returning zest in life, and Francis took up again the
leadership of the gay of Assisi. He started out
on a military expedition but a recurrence of his
disease ended it before he had got beyond a
neighboring town. This marked a spiritual
crisis in his life, for although he gave a banquet
for his companions on his return to Assisi, he
fell into a trance before his guests left. Thence-
forth he was an altered man and dedicated his
life to solitude, prayer, and services to the poor.

He made a pilgrimage to Rome where he
exchanged clothing with a beggar and after
emptying his purse on the altar, experienced
great exaltation in begging before St. Peter's
Cathedral.

On his return to Assisi he passed a leper who
was extremely revolting to Francis. He forced
himself to return and kiss the leper's hands.

This marked the beginning of his services to the lepers and hospitals. He went about in rags, reviled by his former companions who pelted him with mud.

Upon hearing a voice from Heaven which commanded him to rebuild the Chapel of St. Damian, Francis took several bolts of goods from his father's shop which he sold in order to procure money for the reconstruction of the chapel.

His father fearing ultimate ruin at the hands of his impulsive and generous son, took him before the Bishop to disinherit him. Before the legal procedure could be accomplished Francis cast his clothes to his father, saying that he now could truly say "Our Father which art in heaven," and went off singing.

The next three years he spent in the neighborhood of Assisi administering to the poor and the lepers. During mass, at the Chapel of St. Mary of the Angels, the text, Mathew X, 7–10, seemed to apply directly to Francis. Thus in 1209 he started a preaching journey to carry out the precepts of the message. Two fellow townsmen joined him so that they went to Rome and obtained the sanction of Innocent III. This was the beginning of the Franciscan Order.

The zealous work of the disciples throughout Italy started a religious revival among the people. The second order, the order of St. Clara, or the Poor Clares, was the result of a desire of a girl, named Clare, to become a nun governed by the rules of the Franciscan Friars. The third order was for the laity who wished to live under the rules of St. Francis but who could not lead lives dedicated entirely to religion.

Inspired by a desire to preach the gospel to the infidels Francis set out for the Holy Land, but was shipwrecked and had to return to Italy. He then started for Spain to preach to the Moors but again suffered shipwreck. His desire to reach the Holy Land persisted. He made his way to Egypt, where at the battle of Damietta, he was taken prisoner and brought before the sultan. He preached openly to the sultan. He returned to Italy by way of the Holy Land where he gained the foothold that the order has in Palestine today.

On his arrival in Italy he found the government of the order, which had expanded greatly, much confused. Feeling himself inadequate to continue as its head he gave up his authority with the following prayer which is characteristic of his high character and fine sense of justice. "Lord I give thee back this family which Thou didst entrust to me. Thou knowest, most sweet Jesus, that I have no more the powers and the qualities to continue the care of it. I entrust it therefore to the ministers. Let them be responsible before Thee at the Day of Judgment, if any brother by their negligence or their bad example, or by a too severe punishment should go astray."

Two years before his death St. Francis went up to Mount Alverno, in the Apennines, with some of his disciples, and after forty days of fasting and prayer, on the morning of September 14, 1224, a vision appeared to him. After its disappearance St. Francis felt sharp pains mingling with the delight the vision had caused, and upon investigation he saw on his own body the "Stigmata of the Crucified." His long fast and great expenditure of energy resulted in considerable weakness which was so great he had to be carried back to Assisi. He was suffering from advanced tuberculosis.

During his last illness he had one desire after another; first he thought he would like fish, then parsley leaves, until fearing he was asking too much of the Brother who cared for him, he asked to be moved to Portiuncula. He was taken to a hut just outside the Portiuncula Chapel where he died on October 3, 1226, after singing with unusual strength the 141st Psalm of David. On May 25, 1230, he was transferred from his temporary resting place to the beautiful church of St. Francis built by Brother Elias.

Besides being a great evangelist he was also a remarkable writer, being the author of two or three Rules of the Order, the Admonitions and Letters, The Psalms of Praise, and The Prayers, nearly all of them in Latin. In all, there are four Praise Songs, three in Latin and one in Italian. The Italian one is the celebrated Sun Song. His printed writings cover two groups— The Letters and The Rules of the Order. All his writings express the tenderest love of God.

Francis loved God, humanity and Nature greatly. His love was shown in his songs and joyousness. His disciples called themselves the "Lord's minstrels" and Francis constantly admonished them to rejoice in the Lord. His love of humanity, no matter how mean or lowly, is evident from the rules of his order and his insistence on poverty for himself and his disciples. His attitude toward poverty is the subject of some of Dante's poetry and some famous frescos by Giotto. Francis' course has been described thus: "no one has ever set himself to imitate so seriously the life of Christ and to carry out Christ's work in Christ's way." His love of

Nature is best known by his sermon to his "sisters the birds." Even the inanimate aspects of nature, such as the sun and the wind, were the subjects of sermons by him. These are contained in the Fioretti, or the Little Flowers of St. Francis.

His sermons were unusual and of special appeal because they were short admonitions to love the Lord rather than lengthy dissertations on theological precepts. Through his entire life this strain of joyousness is found. During his last illness, in spite of his suffering and the failure of his eyesight, he was cheerful and spent much of his time in song.

On July 16, 1228, Pope Gregory IX canonized Francis. Today, in all parts of the civilized world, we find schools, hospitals, convents and monasteries ruled by the Franciscan Order whose Brothers and Sisters venerate St. Francis as their leader and founder, their patron Saint.

REFERENCES

St. Francis of Assisi. By Johannes Jorgenson.
The Little Flowers; Life and Mirror of St. Francis.
St. Francis of Assisi. By John Tombs. *The Journal of the Outdoor Life*, February, 1923.
Encyclopaedia Brittanica.

FREDERIC CHOPIN

FREDERIC CHOPIN was born in a little Polish village near Warsaw, on February 22, 1810. His father, a Frenchman by birth and a man of education and refinement, devoted much of his time to educational work, becoming, in later life, a professor in three large academies. His mother was an unusual woman whom Frederic spoke of as the "best of mothers." The Chopins were very poor during their early married life, but they did everything possible to create a favorable environment for their children. As a child, Frederic frequently took part in theatrical presentations in celebration of birthdays of his parents and friends. In later life he showed a faculty for mimicry that made his Paris friends predict a successful career on the stage if he had so desired. At one time he assisted his sister in writing a comedy, displaying an unusual comprehension of stage technique which might have been the foundation of a successful opera.

Very early in his life the boy showed great interest in music. As a child he was so susceptible to music and so touched when listening, that it has been said he "wept whenever he heard music, and was with difficulty restrained." He played in public before he was nine. His talent was so evident that his parents decided to do all in their power to promote his musical education. A Bohemian, by the name of Zywny, was employed to teach him piano. Fortunately, he was a teacher who recognized Frederic's unusual originality and gave him opportunity to develop it. With the excellent training he received, it was not long before he was giving concerts and recitals and captivating audiences in his home town. As a result of this local success, of the environment of culture in his own home, of association with his father's pupils who came from families of sound traditions, and of his personal aversion to coarse people, and instinctive avoidance of those lacking in good manners, he found himself, in his early youth, socially recognized by the intellectuals of Poland.

So soon as Frederic showed an interest in musical composition his parents secured the services of a teacher in theory, Joseph Elsner, which proved another fortunate choice. Elsner was not a stereotype teacher. He realized the promise of genius in his exceptional pupil and helped him to develop in his own way. Criticised for this method, Elsner replied: "Leave him alone; he does not follow the common way because his talents are uncommon. He does not adhere to the bold method because he has one of his own and his work will reveal an originality hitherto unknown." It was fortunate that his two teachers guided his early course so wisely; the usual instructor might easily have checked his original tendencies. Frederic learned confidence in these teachers and throughout his life retained a great love and respect for them. In later life, he said: "From Zywny and Elsner even the greatest ass must learn something."

Frederic continued to study and practice most diligently. He frequently would get out of bed during the night and practice, since he always had a piano in his own room. The curiosity of others, particularly of the servants, was aroused by this habit and they would remark, "The poor young gentleman's mind is affected." His general education was provided among his father's private pupils at home, until he entered the Warsaw Lyceum from which he graduated in 1827.

Following graduation his desire to continue the study of music was still paramount. His parents arranged a trip to the great musical centers where he could hear and perhaps meet some of the renowned artists of the day. On the

9th of September, 1828, in his nineteenth year, he set out for Berlin. Soon after his arrival he sent this very interesting letter:

"My Dearly Beloved Parents and Sisters:

"We arrived safely in this big, big city about three o'clock on Sunday afternoon and went direct from the post to the hotel 'Zum Kronprinz,' where we are now. It is a good and comfortable house. The very day we arrived, Professor Jarocki took me to Herr Lichtenstein's, where I met Humboldt. He is not above middle-height; his features cannot be called handsome, but the prominent, broad brow, and the deep penetrating glance reveal the searching intellect of the scholar, who is as great a philanthropist as he is a traveler. He speaks French like his mother tongue; even you would have said so, dear father.

"Herr Lichtenstein promised to introduce me to the first musicians here; and regretted that we had not arrived a few days sooner to have heard his daughter perform at a matinee, last Sunday, with orchestral accompaniments.

"I, for my part, felt but little disappointment; but, whether rightly or wrongly I know not, for I have neither seen nor heard the young lady. The day we arrived there was a performance of 'The Interrupted Sacrifice,' but our visit to

Herr Lichtenstein prevented me from being present.

"Yesterday, the savants had a grand dinner; Herr von Humbolt did not occupy the chair, but a very different looking person, whose name I cannot at this moment recall. However, as he is, no doubt, some celebrity, I have written his name under my portrait of him. I could not refrain from making some caricatures, which I have already classified. The dinner lasted so long that there was not time for me to hear Birnback, the much-praised violinist, of nine years. Today I shall dine alone, having made my excuses to Professor Jarocki, who readily perceived that, to a musician, the performance of such a work as Spontini's 'Ferdinand Cortez,' must be more interesting than an interminable dinner among philosophers. Now I am quite alone, and enjoying a chat with you, my dear ones.

"There is a rumour that the great Paganini is coming here. I only hope it is true. Prince Radziwill is expected on the 20th of this month. It will be a great pleasure to me if he comes. I have, as yet, seen nothing of the Zoölogical Museum, but I know the city pretty well, for I wandered among the beautiful streets also, of the large and decidedly beautiful castle. The chief impression Berlin makes upon me is that of a straggling city which could, I think, contain double its present large population. We wanted to have stayed in the French street, but I am very glad we did not, for it is as broad as our Lezno, and needs ten times as many people as are in it to take off its desolate appearance.

"Today will be my first experience of music in Berlin. Do not think me one sided, dearest Papa, for saying that I would much rather have spent the morning at Schlesinger's than in laboring through the thirteen rooms of the Zoölogical Museum; but I came here for the sake of my musical education, and Schlesinger's library, containing, as it does, the most important musical works of every age and country, is, of course, of more interest to me than any other collection. I console myself with the thought that I shall not miss Schlesinger's and that a young man ought to see all he can, as there is something to be learnt everywhere. This morning I went to Kisting's pianoforte manufactory, at the end of the long Frederic Street, but as there was not a single instrument completed, I had my long walk in vain. Fortunately for me there is a good grand piano in our hotel, which I play on every day, both to my own and the landlord's gratification. . . . "

He remained in Berlin two weeks. On the
return trip he stopped in Zullichau. While
waiting to have the horses changed, an incident,
quoted from Hadden, occurred: "Chopin, thinking of less material things, wandered into one of
the rooms at the inn, and there found a grand
piano. The instrument did not look promis-
ing,—the innkeeper's piano seldom does,—but
appearances are proverbially deceptive. Chopin
rattled off a few arpeggios, and then exclaimed
in delighted surprise; 'O Sancta Cecilia, the
piano is in tune!' The sensation can readily be
imagined, sitting for days in a diligence and then
having a good piano to play upon! Chopin began
to improvise *con amore*. One traveller after
another came and stood around the instrument;
the post-master and his buxom wife followed;
the servants brought up the rear. It reminded
one of Burns' arrival at the wayside hostelries,
when ostlers and everybody else within call
gathered to hear him talk. Chopin became
oblivious to everything, and played on as he
had played at that church service when the
priest made a sudden end of his ecstasy. At
last, when 'the fairies seemed to be singing their
moonlight melodies' and everyone was listening
in rapt attention to 'the elegant arabesques'
sparkling from the musician's fingers, a stentorian

voice called out: 'Gentlemen, the horses are ready.' The listeners looked as if they could strangle the man. 'Confound the disturber!' roared the innkeeper, and the whole company echoed him.

Chopin rose from the instrument, but was implored to go on. 'Stay and play, noble young artist,' cried Boniface. 'I will give you couriers' horses if you will only remain a little longer.' 'Do be persuaded,' insinuated Madame Boniface, who threatened the hesitating player with an embrace. What could Chopin do but resume his improvisation? When he had exhausted himself they brought him wine and cakes, and the women 'filled the pockets of the carriage with the best eatables that the house contained.' One of the company, an old man, went up to Chopin, and 'in a voice trembling with emotion' exclaimed: 'I, too, play the piano, and so know how to appreciate your masterly performance: if Mozart had heard it he would have grasped your hand and cried 'Bravo!' Finally, the landlord seized the musician in his arms and carried him to the conveyance, the postillion growling the while that 'the like of us must climb laboriously on the box by ourselves.' "

In discussing this incident later, Chopin declared that no praise from the press had ever given him so much satisfaction as the homage paid by the German at the inn, "who in his eagerness to hear let his pipe go out."

In slightly less than one month Chopin had returned home. In the following year, 1829, two great artists, Hummel and Paganini came to Warsaw. The experience of meeting and hearing these performers further stimulated Chopin. He decided to go to "The beautiful musical Vienna." After reaching Vienna he wrote: "I am well and in good spirits. Why, I do not know, but the people here are astonished at me; and I wonder at them for finding anything to wonder at in me. I am indebted to good Elsner's letter of recommendation for my exceedingly friendly reception by Herr Haslinger. He did not know how to make me sufficiently welcome; he showed me all the musical novelties he had, made his son play to me, and apologized for not introducing his wife, who had just gone out. In spite of all his politeness, he has not yet printed my compositions. I did not ask him about them, but he said, when showing me one of his finest editions, that my variations on "La ci darem la mano" were to appear next week, in the same style, in *Odeon*. This I certainly had not expected. He strongly advised me to play in public, although it is summer, and therefore not a favorable time for concerts."

As time passed, so many of Vienna's great musicians insisted that Chopin give a concert that he agreed to do so. The concert was a great success. Expressions from press and public were so favorable that he was induced to give a second entertainment. This was even more successful than the first, but he absolutely refused to give a third. Of this he writes: "I only gave a second because I was forced to, and because I thought that people in Warsaw might say: 'He only gave one concert in Vienna, so he could not have been much liked.'" After leaving Vienna he visited Prague, Dresden, and other centers, where he was accorded a great welcome.

Chopin had now envisioned the possibilities that lay beyond his home town. Indeed, he was too much in demand elsewhere. Before leaving home again he fell in love; a circumstance which occurred quite frequently in his life, although he never married. He lacked the courage to speak to his beloved, but he poured out all his passion on paper and played it. The young lady did not return his affection and married another; and Chopin could no longer bear to remain in Warsaw. The regrettable part of the affair was that it seemed to affect Chopin's health and even before he left Warsaw he seemed marked for an early death. He said a sad farewell to his family; his father he saw only once more and his mother never again.

October, 1831, found Chopin in Paris; but before that time he had taken up arms for his country in the revolt against Russia. Warsaw was captured in September, and Chopin now in Paris, poured out his feeling for Poland's fate in the magnificent Etude in C Minor. The question of what he was to do next arose. His reputation as a pianist was established by a concert, in February, 1832, and a second concert added to his fame. He conceived the idea of emigrating to America, but before starting Prince Radziwell took him to a "soiree" at the Rothschilds' where he played so superbly that he was promised several pupils. Chopin was constitutionally unfitted for concert work because of his high strung sensibilities. The teaching of music was more suited to his nature and his popularity in that capacity did not wane until the advent of the Revolution of 1848.

From childhood, Chopin was not strong. He was referred to in childhood, as "a little, frail, delicate, elf of a boy;" and it was said that "the attention of his family was concentrated upon his health." It is well known fact that his family had a history of tuberculosis. In 1826, the same year in which Laennec died of tuberculosis,

Chopin, then only sixteen years old, began to show signs of breaking. His sister, Emilia, was at Reinerz suffering from far advanced tuberculosis. Chopin was sent to stay with her but she died at the age of fourteen while Chopin apparently recovered his usual health.

Today one would not even consider sending a delicate youth to live with a far advanced case of tuberculosis; but the communicability of tuberculosis was not well known then for it was approximately a half century before the discovery of the tubercle bacillus. The painstaking, effective observance of the health measures that we know today should mitigate criticisms of our times by a future generation.

Chopin who has been called the aristocrat of that most aristocratic art, music, found congenial companions in Paris. His list of friends include the names of Meyerbeer, Liszt, Berlioz, Mendelssohn, Heine, George Sand, Countess L'Agault, Cherubisi, Bellini, Balzac and others. His affair with George Sand was the most notable of several. The two geniuses were an absolute contrast in tastes and temperament. They lived in close contact for ten years. It has been claimed that George Sand inspired Chopin to his greatest compositions, and it is also claimed that she broke his heart and was the direct cause of his death. It is impossible to judge, since Chopin said nothing and George Sand said so much that the truth is undiscoverable. The final rupture meant merely the end of an episode to her while it meant the end of life to Chopin.

In 1848 Chopin went to England. He was so weak and racked by his cough that it was most painful to see him, yet when he sat down to the piano his exhaustion seemed to disappear and he played as one inspired. After presentation to the Queen, he played at Court, and then went to Scotland to give recitals. While in Scotland he visited Jane Sterling, who later endowed him with a sum of money which eased somewhat his final days.

Ill and without hope for the future, he returned to Paris, resolved to play no more in public, a resolve he could not fail to keep. In a few short months he was dead. Thus, in 1849, the greatest creative musical genius Poland has ever given to the world was laid to rest in Pere la Chaise at the age of thirty-nine. He was interred in his concert clothes following the Polish custom of burial in uniform, the goblet of Polish earth was emptied over his coffin, and his heart was sent to Warsaw for preservation there.

The greater part of Chopin's fame today rests

on his compositions, which were not popular during his life time. He is said to have revolutionized piano playing by his expert use of the pedals. This method gained him the title of "The poet of the piano." "With Chopin, music was a matter of emotion almost wholly. With him music was always to be free, plastic, and expressive. Emotion was the chief thing with him whether it proved to be dreamy and languorous or fiery and heroic. His sentiment is not sentimentality; his feminine qualities not effeminate. His pathos and intensity are Polish; his etheral delicacy French in style."

REFERENCES

Master Musicians. By J. Cuthbert Hadden.
Elson's Book of Musical Knowledge.

HENRY DAVID THOREAU

I N THE little town of Concord, with a
population then of about two thousand
people, John Thoreau and his wife, Cynthia
Dunbar, lived; and there all their four children
were born. Shortly after Henry was born, on
July 12, 1817, the family moved to Chelmsford
and then to Boston, where Henry's schooling
began. They returned to Concord when he was
six years old and there he lived for the remainder
of his life.

His childhood was a most happy one. John
Thoreau and his wife knew and loved the Concord woods, and took their children to them to
study the birds and flowers. They were poor,
but they made the best of what they had and so
they never felt the pinch of poverty. They
did without tea, coffee, sugar and other luxuries,
that their girls might have the piano their
musical tastes soon proved they needed, and that
a college education might be provided for the
youngest son.

Henry prepared for Harvard University in the
Concord Schools. Even in his boyhood, every
moment outside of school hours was spent with

Nature, exploring all her marvelous wonders. He entered college at the age of sixteen, with the determination to win a scholarship in order to help the serious strain on the family resources. For periods during his college course he taught school, for though it was a comparatively small amount needed to maintain him at Harvard, it meant, nevertheless, much sacrifice on the part of his family.

He was an unusually good student of mathematics and the classics, but instead of bending all his efforts to obtaining honors in these studies, he deliberately devoted much of his time to the college library, an opportunity to the country boy not to be neglected. He acquired the widespread knowledge of authors that was ever remarkable. He received the degree of Bachelor of Arts in 1837, without honors, but with an excellent fund of information not usually included in a college course.

The natural field open to a youth fresh from college was teaching and, for lack of a better opportunity, Thoreau took charge of the town-school in Concord. This service was of short duration, since he refused to administer corporal chastisement and since the town did not feel that it was getting its money's worth without it. So he whipped six scholars and then resigned to find a place where such methods were not required.

The next year, with his adored brother, John, he took a position in the Concord Academy, and made of it a great success. John was the principal, while Henry had charge of the classical department. The scholars, in later life, remembered both brothers with affection and gratitude for the breadth and the quality of their instruction. The two were enough unlike to increase the interest and happiness of their relationship. During a summer vacation together on the river, John died very suddenly from lockjaw, resulting from a seemingly trifling cut received while shaving. The shock completely overwhelmed Henry, who for a long time was helpless and inconsolable.

At length, Thoreau recovered his poise, but it seemed as though a part of himself had been torn away. He turned instinctively to Nature for healing and spent many hours in the woods. In the next few years he worked with his father in the pencil-making business. Thanks to Henry's persistence and careful study of the subject, the Thoreaus began the manufacture of a pencil similar to the good German sort, replacing the hard, gritty, inefficient leads then made in America.

In the year 1849 the process of electrotyping was invented in Boston. The man engaged in the business wanted the best lead available. Consequently he ordered the lead from John Thoreau, who guarded his method of making it very carefully. This increased their business materially, and eventually the making of lead for electrotypes became their principal trade, with the pencils as a mere side-line.

As soon as the business was on its way to prosperity Thoreau resigned his partnership with his father. He had few wants; plain food, strong clothing and a telescope sufficed. He was a good gardener, mechanic, and emergency man, and he did all sorts of odd jobs both at home and among his friends. He wrote articles for magazines, which brought him little money, and books then hardly salable. Today they are esteemed as classics. His leading profession was that of land surveyor, and the farther it led him into the woods and fields the more he enjoyed it.

It is through his two year's encampment, on the shore of a small lake in the Walden Woods, a mile or so south of Concord, that Thoreau is best known to the world. His hermit-life was not a protest against the luxury and restraint of society, nor a strict discipline of the soul imposed upon himself after the fashion of monks and saints. He went there to live a life of labor and study, free from interruption, and when he had exhausted the advantages of his solitude he left it. He edited his first book and satisfied himself that he was fit to be an author. The events and the thoughts of his life at Walden may be read in his book under that name.

The years he spent there were happy, wholesome years, expanding his whole future by their teaching. He left his retreat frequently, for his family were a little anxious and troubled for him, fearing the hardship and danger of his life at Walden. He came home often to see them and to help about the garden and the house, or to drop in at other friendly homes. While at Walden, the episode of his refusal to pay his poll-tax occurred. The slave-power had forced upon the country the war of invasion with Mexico. Ordinarily a good citizen, he felt that the government had sunk so low that the time had come for a rebellion of his own. When the town constable, himself a good friend, came to arrest him, he offered to pay Thoreau's tax for him, not understanding that his refusal was a matter of principle rather than of poverty. He spent a night in jail and, after dark, some unrecognized person left the tax money at the constable's door; whereupon, the next morning that worthy gentleman gladly sent Thoreau away.

Thoreau did not seek to be drawn into the question of slavery, but it came to his cabin door. He solved it as he felt right. He sheltered the fugitive slave, helped and guided him and others; later on becoming one of the managers of the Undergrown Railroad. Thoreau did not neglect his civic duties, in spite of the tax episode. He was aroused by the low moral tone of the county and, again and again, he left the quiet of the woods to speak in Concord and elsewhere for freedom of person, thought and conscience.

Music was his early and lifelong friend. His sisters made the home full of it; and the sweet tunes of Mrs. Hawthorne's music-box comforted him much in the lonely days after John's death. The songs of the birds were his sweetest music, and many a girl and boy owes to him the opening of a gate to almost fairy knowledge of the voices often unknown and unnoted by others.

His friends were many,—their names known to all the world. He was often at the home of the Emersons and early formed deep and lasting friendships with Ellery Channing, Alcott, Hawthorne, Margaret Fuller and Horace Greeley. He was acquainted with Daniel Webster and Walt Whitman, both of whom visited Concord. Ellery Channing, who perhaps knew him more intimately than anyone else, said: "In his own home he was one of those characters who may be called 'household treasures;' always on the spot, with skillful eye and hand, to raise the best melons in the garden, plant the orchard with choicest trees, or act as extempore mechanic; fond of the pets, his sister's flowers, or sacred Tabby; kittens were his favorites; he would play with them by the half-hour. No whim or coldness, no absorption of his time by public or private business, deprived those to whom he belonged of his kindness and affection. He did the duties that lay nearest, and satisfied those in his immediate circle; and whatever the impression from the theoretical part of his writings, when the matter is probed to the bottom, good sense and good feeling will be detected in it."

Thoreau was but forty-four years old when he died. He contracted a chill by long stooping, in a wet snow storm, engaged in counting the growth-rings on some old tree stumps. His tuberculosis became active. He lived a year and a half after this exposure and made a trip to Minnesota in the vain search for health. His reasons for going to Minnesota are brought out in the letters written by Thoreau to Harrison Blake:

"Mr. Blake,—I am still as much an invalid as when you and Brown were here, if not more of one, and at this rate there is danger that the cold weather may come again, before I get over my bronchitis. The doctor accordingly tells me that I must 'clear out' to the West Indies, or elsewhere,—he does not seem to care much where. But I decided against the West Indies, on account of their muggy heat in the summer, and the South of Europe, on account of the expense of time and money, and have at last concluded that it will be most expedient for me to try the air of Minnesota, say somewhere about St. Paul. I am only waiting to be well enough to start. Hope to get off within a week or ten days.

"The inland air may help me at once, or it may not. At any rate, I am so much of an invalid, that I shall have to study my comfort in traveling to a remarkable degree,—stopping to rest, etc., etc., if need be. I think to get a through ticket to Chicago, with liberty to stop frequently on the way, making my first stop of consequence at Niagara Falls, several days or a week, at a private boarding-house; then a night or day at Detroit; and as much at Chicago as my health may require. At Chicago I can decide at what point (Fulton, Dunleith, or another) to strike the Mississippi and take a boat to St. Paul.

"I trust to find a private boarding-house in one or various agreeable places in that region and spend my time there. I expect, and shall be prepared to be gone three months; and I would like to return by a different route, perhaps Mackinaw and Montreal.

"I have thought of finding a companion, of course, yet not seriously; because I had no right to offer myself as a companion to anybody, having such a peculiarly private and all-absorbing but miserable business as my health, and not altogether this, to attend to, causing me to stop here and go there, etc., etc., unaccountably.

"Nevertheless, I have just now decided to let you know of my intention, thinking it barely possible that you might like to make a part or the whole of this journey at the same time, and that perhaps your own health may be such as to be benefited by it.

"Pray let me know if such a statement offers any temptations to you. I write in great haste for the mail, and must omit all the moral."

After reaching Minnesota, he wrote the following letter to F. B. Sanborn: "Mr. Sanborn,—I was very glad to find awaiting me, on my arrival here, on Sunday afternoon, a letter from you.

I have performed this journey in a very dead and alive manner, but nothing has come so near waking me up as the receipt of letters from Concord. I read yours, and one from my sister, (and Horace Mann, his four), near the top of a remarkable isolated bluff here, called Barn Bluff, or the Grange, or Redwing Bluff, some four hundred and fifty feet high, and half a mile long,—a bit of the main bluff or bank standing alone. The top, as you know, rises to the general level of the surrounding country, the river having eaten out so much. Yet the valley just above and below this, (we are at the head of Lake Pepin), must be three or four miles wide.

"I am not even so well informed as to the progress of the war as you suppose. I have seen but one Eastern paper, (that, by the way, was the *Tribune*), for five weeks. I have not taken much pains to get them; but, necessarily, I have not seen any paper at all for more than a week at a time. The people of Minnesota have seemed to me more cold,—to feel less implicated in this war than the people of Massachusetts. It is apparent that Massachusetts, for one State at least, is doing much more than her share in carrying it on. However, I have dealt partly with those of Southern birth, and have seen but a little way beneath the surface. I was glad to be told yesterday that there was a good deal of weeping here at Redwing the other day, when the volunteers stationed at Fort Snelling followed the regulars to the seat of the war. They do not weep when their children go up the river to occupy the deserted forts, though they may have to fight the Indians there.

"I do not even know what the attitude of England is at present.

"The grand feature hereabouts is, of course, the Mississippi River. Too much can hardly be said of its grandeur, and of the beauty of this portion of it, (from Dunleith, and probably from Rock Island to this place). St. Paul is a dozen miles below the Falls of St. Anthony, or near the head of uninterrupted navigation on the main stream, about two thousand miles from its mouth. There is not a 'rip' below that, and the river is almost as wide in the upper as the lower part of its course. Steamers go up to the Sauk Rapids, above the Falls, near a hundred miles farther, and then you are fairly in the pinewoods and lumbering country. Thus it flows from the pine to the palm.

"The lumber, as you know, is sawed chiefly at the Falls of St. Anthony, (what is not rafted in the log to ports far below), having given rise to the towns of St. Anthony, Minneapolis, etc., etc. In coming up the river from Dunleith, you meet with great rafts of sawed lumber and of logs, twenty rods or more in length, by five or six wide, floating down, all from the pine region above the Falls. An old Maine lumberer, who has followed the same business here, tells me that the sources of the Mississippi were comparatively free from rocks and rapids, making easy work for them; but he thought that the timber was more knotty here than in Maine.

"It has chanced that about half the men whom I have spoken with in Minnesota, whether travelers or settlers, were from Massachusetts.

"After spending some three weeks in and about St. Paul, St. Anthony, and Minneapolis, we made an excursion in a steamer, some three hundred or more miles up the Minnesota, (St. Peter's) River, to Redwood, or the Lower Sioux Agency, in order to see the plains and the Sioux, who were to receive their annual payment there. This is eminently the river of Minnesota, (for she shares the Mississippi with Wisconsin), and it is of incalculable value to her. It flows through a very fertile country, destined to be famous for its wheat; but it is a remarkably winding stream, so that Redwood is only half as far from its mouth by land as by water. There was not a straight reach a mile in length as far as we went,—generally you could not see a quarter of a mile of water, and the boat was steadily turning this way or that. At the greater bends, as the Traverse des Sioux, some of the passengers were landed, and walked across to be taken in on the other side. Two or three times you could have thrown a stone across the neck of the isthmus, while it was from one to three miles around it. It was a very novel kind of navigation to me. The boat was perhaps the largest that had been up so high, and the water was rather low, (it had been about fifteen feet higher). In making a short turn, we repeatedly and designedly ran square into the steep and soft bank, taking in a cart-load of earth,—this being more effectual than the rudder to fetch us about again; or the deeper water was so narrow and close to the shore, that we were obliged to run into and break down at least fifty trees which overhung the water, when we did not cut them off, repeatedly losing a part of our outworks, though the most exposed had been taken in. I could pluck almost any plant on the bank from the boat. We very frequently got aground, and then drew ourselves along with a windlass and a cable fastened to a tree, or we swung round in the current and completely blocked up and blockaded the river, one end of the boat resting on each shore. And yet we would haul ourselves round again with the windlass and cable in an hour or two, though the boat was about one hundred and sixty feet long, and drew some three feet of water, or, often, water and sand. It was one consolation to know that in such a case we were all the while damming the river, and so raising it. We once ran fairly on to a concealed rock, with a shock that aroused all the passengers, and rested there, and the mate went below with a lamp, expecting to find a hole, but he did not. Snags and sawyers were so common that I forgot to mention them. The sound of the boat rumbling over one was the ordinary music. However, as long as the boiler did not burst, we knew that no serious accident was likely to happen. Yet this is a singularly navigable river, more so than the Mississippi above the Falls, and it is owing to its very crookedness. Ditch it straight, and it would not only be very swift, but soon run out. It was from ten to fifteen rods wide near the mouth, and from eight to ten or twelve at Redwood. Though the current was swift, I did not see a 'rip' on it, and only three or four rocks. For three months in the year I am told that it can be navigated by small steamers about twice as far as we went, or to its source in Big Stone Lake; and a former Indian agent told me that at high water it was thought that such a steamer might pass into the Red River.

"In short, this river proved so very long and navigable, that I was reminded of the last letter or two in the voyage of the Baron la Hontan, (written near the end of the seventeenth century, I think), in which he states, that, after reaching the Mississippi (by the Illinois or Wisconsin), the limit of previous exploration westward, he voyaged up it with his Indians, and at length turned up a great river coming in from the west, which he called "La Riviere Longue;" and he relates various improbable things about the country and its inhabitants, so that this letter has been regarded as pure fiction, or, more properly speaking, a lie. But I am somewhat inclined now to reconsider the matter.

"The Governor of Minnesota, (Ramsay), the superintendent of Indian affairs in this quarter, and the newly-appointed Indian Agent were on board; also a German band from St. Paul, a small cannon for salutes, and the money for the Indians, (ay, and the gamblers, it was said, who were to bring it back in another boat). There were about one hundred passengers, chiefly from St. Paul, and more or less recently from the northeastern States; also half a dozen young educated Englishmen. Chancing to speak with one who sat next to me, when the voyage was nearly half over, I found that he was the son of the Rev. Samuel May, and a class-mate of yours, and had been looking for us at St. Anthony.

"The last of the little settlements on the river was New Ulm, about one hundred miles this side of Redwood. It consists wholly of Germans. We left them one hundred barrels of salt, which will be worth something more, when the water is lowest, than at present.

"Redwood is a mere locality,—scarcely an Indian village,—where there is a store, and some houses have been built for them. We were now fairly on the great plains, and looking south; and, after walking that way three miles, could see no tree in that horizon. The buffalo were said to be feeding within twenty-five or thirty miles.

"A regular council was held with the Indians, who had come in on their ponies, and speeches were made on both sides through an interpreter, quite in the described mode,—the Indians, as usual, having the advantage in point of truth and earnestness, and therefore eloquence. The most prominent chief was named Little Crow. They were quite dissatisfied with the white man's treatment of them, and probably have reason to be so. This council was to be continued for two or three days,—the payment to be made the second day; and another payment to other hands a little higher up, on the Yellow Medicine, (a tributary of the Minnesota), a few days thereafter.

"In the afternoon, the half-naked Indians performed a dance, at the request of the Governor, for our amusement and their own benefit; and then we took leave of them, and of the officials who had come to treat with them.

"Excuse these pencil marks, but my inkstand is unscrewable, and I can only direct my letter at the bar. I could tell you more, and perhaps more interesting things, if I had time. I am considerably better than when I left home, but still far from well.

"Our faces are already set toward home. Will you please let my sister know that we shall probably start for Milwaukee 'and Mackinaw in a day or two, (or as soon as we hear from home), via Prairie du Chien, and not LaCrosse.

"I am glad to hear that you have written to Cholmondeley, as it relieves me of some responsibility."

After returning from Minnestoa to Concord, Thoreau wrote to Daniel Ricketson as follows:

"Friend Ricketson,—When your last letter was written I was away in the far Northwest, in search of health. My cold turned to bronchitis, which made me a close prisoner almost up to the moment of my starting on that journey, early in May. As I had an incessant cough, my doctor told me that I must 'clear out,'—to the West Indies, or elsewhere,—so I selected Minnesota. I returned a few weeks ago, after a good deal of steady traveling, considerably, yet not essentially, better; my cough still continuing. If I don't mend very quickly, I shall be obliged to go to another climate again very soon.

"My ordinary pursuits, both indoors and out, have been for the most part omitted, or seriously interrupted,—walking, boating, scribbling, etc. Indeed, I have been sick so long that I have almost forgotten what it is to be well; and yet I feel that it is in all respects only my envelope. Channing and Emerson are as well as usual; but Alcott, I am sorry to say, has for some time been more or less confined by a lameness, perhaps of a neuralgic character, occasioned by carrying too great a weight on his back while gardening.

"On returning home, I found various letters awaiting me; among others, one from Cholmondeley, and one from yourself.

"Of course I am sufficiently surprised to hear of your conversion; yet I scarcely know what to say about it, unless that, judging by your account, it appears to me a change which concerns yourself peculiarly, and will not make you more valuable to mankind. However, perhaps I must see you before I can judge.

"Remembering your numerous invitations, I write this short note now, chiefly to say that, if you are to be at home, and it will be quite agreeable to you, I will pay you a visit next week, and take such rides or sauntering walks with you as an invalid may."

About two months later he wrote Daniel Ricketson again. In mentioning his health and treatment he said: "I think that, on the whole, my health is better than when you were here; but my faith in the doctors has not increased. . . . Instead of riding on horseback, I ride in a wagon about every day."

The last months he was confined to the house, but he was very brave and worked on his manuscript, until the end. A Calvinistic aunt, coming to see him, asked, "Henry, have you made your peace with God?" and the pleasant answer came, "I did not know we had ever quarreled, Aunt."

On December 19th, Thoreau's sister, Sophia,

wrote a letter for him, replying to one from Daniel Ricketson. She said: "The air and exercise which he enjoyed during the fine autumn days were a benefit to him; he seemed stronger, had a good appetite, and was able to attend somewhat to his writings; but since the cold weather has come, his cough has increased and he is able to go out but seldom. Just now he is suffering from an attack of pleurisy, which confines him wholly to the house. His spirits do not fail him; he continues in his usual serene mood, which is very pleasant for his friends as well as himself. I am hoping for a short winter and early spring, that the invalid may again be out-of-doors."

The following is the last letter Thoreau ever wrote. He dictated it to his sister, in reply to a letter received from Myron Benton, in which Benton complimented him very highly on two of his books, "Week" and "Walden."

"Dear Sir: I thank you for your very kind letter, which, ever since I received it, I have intended to answer before I died, however briefly. I am encouraged to know, that, so far as you are concerned, I have not written my books in vain. I was particularly gratified, some years ago, when one of my friends and neighbors said, 'I wish you would write another book,—

write it for me.' He is actually more familiar with what I have written than I am myself.

"The verses you refer to, in Conway's *Dial*, were written by F. B. Sanborn, of this town. I never wrote for that journal.

"I am pleased when you say that in *The Week* you like especially 'those little snatches of poetry interspersed through the book,' for these, I suppose, are the least attractive to most readers. I have not been engaged in any particular work on Botany, or the like, though, if I were to live, I should have much to report on Natural History generally.

"You ask particularly after my health. I suppose that I have not many months to live; but, of course, I know nothing about it. I may add that I am enjoying existence as much as ever, and regret nothing.

                              "Yours truly,
                              "Henry D. Thoreau,
                              "by Sophia E. Thoreau."

Thoreau died on May 6, 1862, and was buried in the village cemetery, "Sleepy Hollow," where many of his famous friends now lie beside him. Said one of them: "With Thoreau's life something went out of the Concord woods and fields and river that will never return. He so loved

Nature, delighted in her every aspect, that he seemed to infuse himself into her."

REFERENCES

Henry Thoreau: As Remembered by a Young Friend. By Edward Waldo Emerson.
Henry Thoreau. American Men of Letters Series. By F. B. Sanborn.
The Life of Henry David Thoreau. By F. B. Sanborn.
Henry David Thoreau. Stories of Authors. By Edwin Watts Chubb.

FEDOR DOSTOIEVSKY

THE name of Dostoievsky is usually linked with those of Tolstoy and Puskin. His works are not finished and polished master-pieces, yet they "anticipated in a remarkable manner some of the conspicuous tenets of his great successor, Tolstoy." Dostoievsky seldom had the time to rewrite and polish his books, for with the possible exception of two, they were written under the urgent need of money, to keep his wife and children from starving. Added to this pecuniary problem, Dostoievsky was suffer-ing from chronic tuberculosis and epilepsy.

He is unequaled in his ability to make one love and suffer with the characters in his works. Even as life tortured Dostoievsky's characters, so it tortured Dostoievsky himself, and made him look upon existence as a thing of awful gravity and perpetual difficulty. Since poverty, cold and hunger were so often his lot, it is no wonder that he was a master at describing the holes and corners where poverty and wretched-ness fester. He insisted that man seeks suffer-ing, and loves it, and needs it as much as he does material happiness. This is the essence of his "doctrine of purification by suffering—by suffering alone." Broken in health and spirit he gave way frequently to periods of great despair and bitterness until his outlook on life was distorted.

Dostoievsky was born in the work-house hospital in Moscow, on October 21, 1821, where his father was a staff physician. He was the second son of a large family. His father never possessed means beyond his meagre salary, and the whole family resided in a tiny three-room official flat. Later, the family acquired a small piece of property out in the province of Tula, where they moved in the summer time and where a little variety crept into their lives. Their diversions were very few, but the change of scene and the new impressions of country life were welcome. Their father was very strict, disliking to see them at play, anxious to have them always at work. The children were never petted or indulged, but urged to a disciplined, discreet mode of life which stressed the performance of duty. The father stinted himself that his children might have a good education and demanded in return a total abstinence from all frivolity. In the country the children had a little more freedom, for they were constantly in the open air, watching and supervising the labors

of the peasants in the fields. Feodor preferred
to talk with the workers rather than play with
his brothers. The saddest day in the lives of
the Dostoievsky family came when the news
reached them that the little country home had
burned to the ground.

Their education was begun very early and as
soon as the boys were old enough they were sent
to a school kept by Tchermak in Moscow.
Though Dostoievsky wanted to give his children
the best education possible, it was eccentric in
method and over-strict in form. Up to the age
of sixteen, the children were treated like infants.
They were never allowed out-of-doors alone or
allowed any pocket money. Reared exclusively
in the family circle, without other companions,
they were entirely ignorant of life beyond the
hospital walls. So strict was the father's rule
that he inspired awe rather than affection. He
never ceased to instill into his children the idea
that life was a hard and difficult task, wherein
even the smallest mistake may eventually spell
ruin. Upon a nervous, impressionable child
such as Dostoievsky, this regime was bound to
exercise a harmful influence. From earliest
childhood, he fell into the habit of shrinking from
life, and there appeared in him that diffident
suspicious attitude towards himself and others

which ended in wrecking his later years. Yet his boyhood was the happiest period of his existence, for the family life, though monotonous, was peaceful.

Dostoievsky read extensively, but it was most irregular reading; for he read anything and everything he could lay hands on, novels and poetry especially. This formless reading developed and humanized Dostoievsky's talent, but it over-enriched an already fertile imagination which needed a course of discipline.

Early in 1837, Dostoievsky's mother died of tuberculosis and the father decided to send his sons to the School of Engineering in St. Petersburg. Mikhail, his brother, of whom he was very fond, was rejected, so he entered alone; alone he remained, since he held himself aloof from his companions. He worked diligently, but without enthusiasm. From dissipation of any kind he turned with absolute loathing. His mental condition became truly pitiful, while money difficulties made him very irritable, and he dared not write to his father for money except for the barest necessities.

In 1839, his father died and, in 1843, his course completed, Dostoievsky entered the Service proper. His pecuniary troubles continued to be as troublesome as before—not because he was now so much in need of money, but that he was so impractical and money slipped through his hands like water. Though his lack of funds worried him, he had neither the will nor the power to exercise self-denial. To the end of his life he never learned to make both ends meet.

He left the Service after a year and took to literature. In the beginning he tried his hand at translations and later completed an unfinished novel. Neither of these ever saw the light of day, but at the same time he had begun his first independent work, "Poor Folk," the only novel which he ever had time to elaborate or rewrite. The problem of how to publish it disturbed him for a bit, but through a friend it was finally placed in the hands of a publisher, who sat up all night to read it and proclaimed it a masterpiece. The glory which resulted seemed to turn his head and he was prone to exaggerate his success. He found himself in a literary circle composed of the best men of the period, but not for long did he remain there. Dazed with his sudden and brilliant entry into the literary world, he could not conceal his triumph and showed that he considered himself far superior to his companions. Some of them took to leading him on for the sake of seeing him trip himself up. To anyone as nervous and suspicious as Dostoievsky, this was fatal; for his rage rendered him unconscious of what he was saying. Sure that they were trying jealously to belittle his talent, he withdrew from the circle, saying he no longer desired to be acquainted with men of such grudging natures.

A few failures, following "Poor Folk," speedily showed him that he was not the genius he imagined himself to be, and plunged him more deeply into debt. Frantic, he undertook more literary work than his strength could possibly stand. His physical health was poor and his mental state was now almost bordering on insanity. He became very despondent and felt inclined to believe in the current opinion that he had written himself out.

In this frame of mind and body, it was inevitable that Dostoievsky should become a member of one of the revolutionary circles then rapidly spreading and eventually he was arrested and thrown into prison. During the first stage of his prison life in Russia, he was not greatly dismayed by his surroundings or troubled about his future. He read a great deal, planned two novels and some short stories, and seemed not to suffer much. Finally, he received the notice of his death sentence, and was led out with thirty others and lined up against the wall before the firing squad. Within a minute of the order to fire, word came that the death sentence had been commuted to four years of penal servitude in Siberia. This was a terrible experience, so terrible that one of the men actually went mad.

Here began a life full of privation, for the prison conditions were frightful, and Dostoievsky was suffering from repeated hemorrhages and pains in his chest. He experienced tortures from the poor food and the unbearable cold. The little money his brother was able to send him brought him a few luxuries in the way of food supplies, but he longed for books and none were allowed except the Bible. His companions were, for the most part, criminals of the lowest order from whom he instinctively shrank; and as they too hated him because he was not of their kind, he had no choice but to live within himself, dwelling on his past memories. It seems impossible that a man could have received any benefit from such an experience, yet undoubtedly he did. Up to the time of his arrest his mental condition was deplorable and might easily have led to suicide. He had taken up arms against life. But during four years in prison he had time to reconstruct his whole life and to realize the futility of battling against existing conditions.

Released in March, 1854, he became a private in the Siberian Corps; but in October he was promoted to the rank of ensign and allowed to retire. Not until then was he able to resume his literary activities and he immediately brought forth the famous "Letters from a Dead House," based on his own prison experiences.

While still in Siberia, after his term of penal servitude, although utterly destitute he married a Russian lady of as uncertain a disposition as himself. Undoubtedly their domestic life was as stormy as it was brief. His wife died a few years after their marriage from tuberculosis.

Back in St. Petersburg, he published, in conjunction with his brother, for the space of two years, a journal known as *Vremya*, which in the beginning enjoyed considerable success. Dostoievsky acted both as editor and contributor and in both capacities he worked strenuously. "The Fateful Question," an article by a fellow contributor, was settled by the Censorship in the suppression of the *Vremya*. The brothers attempted to continue publication under another title, but the subscribers had fallen off and they were deeply in debt. Added to these misfortunes, the brother died three months later, leaving his wife and children destitute. Dostoievsky, in desperation, began another novel, written as he said,

"Under the lash of necessity and against time."
Then began a period of great novel writing when
with spasmodic activity, he produced a mass of
hastily written material in which his unequaled
genius appears only in fitful gleams. During
this time he wrote "Crime and Punishment,"
his greatest novel and perhaps the best known
in America. In no other work does he show
such depth of analysis or such marvellously
artistic skill. In this work he frequently im-
presses the reader with the fact that in every
life, no matter how degraded, a bright flame of
good keeps burning.

Despite the fact that he received a great deal
of money for his novel, most of it was spent in
payment of debts incurred during the publication of the journal, and he remained as poor as
ever. He made the mistake of binding himself
to one publisher, under contract to produce
another novel by a certain date. In order to
facilitate his work he hired a stenographer
who very shortly afterwards became his second
wife.

The next four years were spent abroad mostly
in Germany and Switzerland, in order to escape
his creditors. His lack of funds remained as
chronic as ever, and he frequently had to sell
articles of his own or his wife's clothing to pay

for their meager existence. He complained of illness, but he worked almost continuously, producing a novel a year.

In 1871, Dostoievsky and his wife returned to St. Petersburg, and his financial circumstances improved. He became the editor of *The Citizen* on a salary, with additional fees for extra articles. His wife obtained better terms for the publication of his existing works, which brought him an annual income of several thousand roubles. He began the *Diary of a Writer* and with every issue his fame grew, until it was impossible to supply the demand.

He became seriously ill just ten days before his death, the fatal issue resulting from a hemorrhage. He died on January 28, 1881. His funeral pageant was such a one as had never been seen in Russia before, more than forty thousand people coming from far and near to do honor to him.

Although for the greater part of his life Dostoievsky was in poverty and suffering from two chronic maladies—tuberculosis and epilepsy, yet critics say of him that he is not only the greatest of all Russian novelists, but also one of the greatest writers the world has ever produced. His works are acclaimed today because of their marvelous fidelity to the principles of abnormal psychology—a science that was almost unheard of in Dostoievsky's time.

REFERENCES

Dostoievsky: His Life and Literary Activity. By Evgenii Solovev.
Letters of Dostoievsky. Translated by C. E. Mayne.
Feodor Mikhailovich Dostoievsky. By John Tombs. *The Journal of the Outdoor Life*, April, 1923.

ARTEMUS WARD

CHARLES FARRAR BROWNE was born at Waterford, Maine, on April 26, 1834. His mother was Caroline Eliza Farrar, and his father, Levi Browne. The latter was very public spirited and held several public offices. Besides running a farm and a store he was engaged in surveying.

Charles was not an exceptional student, but was clever in recitations and very popular in "getting up a show." One of his boyhood pranks was to assist a number of play fellows to lock in the school-house as many hens as they could catch on a Sunday night in the village. The boys enjoyed two extra days vacation as a result.

When Charles was thirteen years old his father died. This made it necessary for him to begin work. He had some desire to take up printing, since his brother, Cyrus, seven years his senior, was already engaged in that trade. Consequently he took the stage to Lancaster, New Hampshire, where he was to learn the trade in the office of the *Weekly Democrat*. He lived with Mr. John M. Rix, publisher of the paper.

The young man was of so gawky an appearance that the cook in Mr. Rix's family, on seeing him, remarked: "I guess we've got a queer kind of critter this time, but I bet he can eat." When asked by the children how she intended to feed him, the cook replied: "We'll fill him up with green apples."

As an apprentice, he was often sent about the country to collect bills from the farmers; and Mr. Rix's fifteen-year-old daughter was often sent along to see that he worked. Her observations led to the statement, in later years, that "He would rather talk to the people and tell stories than ask them for money." The printing office was over a room stored to the ceiling with barrels filled with rum. The boys had drilled a hole through the floor and into one of the barrels, then, with a long tube they would drink their fill. This occasionally led to considerable disorder and on one occasion it became so bad that the shop could not be used for a week. This time they were all discharged.

Upon his return home, after about a year's experience in the print shop, Charles told his mother that his education was insufficient for success as a printer. He then entered the Norway Liberal Institute which was located in Norway, a town near Waterford, and secured a position with *The Norway Advertiser*. In the Institute, as in his earlier days, he did no out-standing school work, but he took great interest in the debates and the journalistic activities of the school. While a debate was in session, he usually occupied one of the three chairs on the platform, and it is said that "he would tilt the chair back against the wall, cross his legs, with his boots much in evidence, and loll in this attitude until his turn came in the discussion, when he easily took the lead in skill and wit as a debater. The drawl that gave charm to his speech was already there, and his cleverness drew large audiences to the school hall, the town always turning out when it knew that 'Charley' was to talk."

After the failure of *The Norway Advertiser*, he worked consecutively for *The Standard* of New Bedford, *The News*, of Fall River and *The Skowhegan Clarion*, of Augusta. He disliked this place very much and one night let himself down by a bell-cord from a second story window and returned to his home. Later, he secured a position in Boston, where he remained three years. During this period he prepared his first manuscript for publication. He wrote of a Fourth of July celebration he had witnessed long before. He sent the manuscript in anonymously. It was a happy day when he saw his article in print. He celebrated the appearance of his article in print by a night at the theater. Of this he later said: "Had a good time of it and thought I was the greatest man in Boston."

With all his worldly possessions, Charles left Boston with Ohio as his destination. He found employment for a week in a little Kentucky school; but since he was not robust enough to handle the big boys who believed in testing out the teacher's muscle, he decided that teaching was not what he desired to do and departed without waiting for his pay.

His next position was on the *Seneca Advertiser* of Tiffen, Ohio, where he remained for a year. In Toledo he was local editor of *The Toledo Commercial* from which he went to *The Cleveland Plain Dealer* as city editor at ten dollars a week. The fortunes of *The Dealer* began to improve under Browne. He made friends easily and was always cheerful and full of humor and quick wit. On January 30, 1858, the first communication from the hand of "Artemus Ward" appeared in the form of a crude, misspelled, but exceedingly funny letter, purporting to be from one Artemus Ward, a proprietor of a side-show, then in Pittsburg.

The idea caught popular fancy and other

letters from the showman were eagerly awaited.
The letters continued to appear, from time to
time, as the showman moved from one town to
another with his extraordinary show. In his
letters "Mr. Ward" gave vivid descriptions of
local events and lengthy discussions on world
news in general. The letters went on for about
two years, and have been compiled in one volume
known as "Artemus Ward—His Book." A few
of the letters from *The Plain Dealer* follow:

"A LETTER FROM A SIDE-SHOWMAN

"Mr. Artemus Ward, proprietor of the well-
known side-show, writes us from Pittsburg as
follows:

"'Pittsburg, Jan. 27, 18 & 58
"'The Plane Deeler:
"'Sir:
"'i write to no how about the show bisnes in
Cleeveland i have a show consisting in part of a
Calforny Bare two snakes tame foxies &c also
wax works my wax works is hard to beat, all
say they is life and nateral curiosities among my
wax works is Our Saveyer Gen. taylor and
Docktor Webster in the ackt of killing Parkman.
now mr. Editor scratch off few lines and tel me
how is the show bisnes in your good city i shal
have hanbils printed at your offis you scratch

my back and i will scratch your back, also git up a grate blow in the paper about my show don't forgit the wax works.

            " 'Yours truly,

                Artemus Ward

                    Pitsburg Penny.

" 'p S pitsburg is a I horse town.   A.W'

"We believe Mr. W. would do well with his show here, and advise him to come along immediately."

           " 'Wheeling, va feby the 3 18&58

" 'Gents—ime movin sloly down your way i want you should git up a tremendus excitement in the columz of your valerble paper about my show.   it nox the socks off from all other shows in the u.s. my wax works is the delight of all. the papers sets my works up steep.   i want the editers to cum to my show Free as the flours of may, but I Dont want them to ride a Free hos to deth.   The Editers in pittsburg air the sneakinest cusses i ever see.   they Come to the Show in krowds and then ask me ten Sents a line for pufs. they said if i made a Row or Disturbence abowt it they would all jine in angiv my wax works perfeck Hel.   the editer of the journal said he would Tip over my apel cart in duble quick time, if i Blowed round him about hi prises.   i put up to ther Extorshuns long Enough & left in

[156]

Dizgust. now which papers is the most respectful in your city. i shal get my hanbils printed at your offis—i want you to understan that, but i must keep the other papers in good umer. now mr. Ed tel me franckly without no disception for disception off all kinds i do dispise. Also git up a excitement in the Plane Deeler sinse i last wrote you ive Added A Cangeroo two my collecksion of Living Wild Beasts. it would make you larf to see the little cuss jump and squeal. if you say anything abowt my show pleas state my snakes is under perfeck subjecshun.   " 'yours truly,

A. Ward.
" 'p.S.—my wax works is hard to beet.' "

"Letter from Artemus Ward—The proprietor of the well-known Side Show writes us again:

        " 'Kolumbus ohio Febey the 16 18&58
" 'Gents—here i am in the kapertal sity of Ohio. ime gradualy gitting down yr way. as the Poit says, ime on the Winding way mr. Editer. i gut shaimfully uzed up to whealin by a nusepaper. i calls no names but theres a editer in whealin whose meaner than biled vittles. he cums to my show every Night and sets it up Steap in his nusepaper and calls me the erbane an Inderfatergerble Ward, but when i stops

gittin my Hanbils struck off up to his offis the pussylanermus cuss changis his toon an abuses me worse nor a injun. he blowed up my wax works and called me a horery heded itinerunt vagerbone. but let it pas. ive bun in the Show Bisness now goin on 22 years and my hed is frostid ore with white and ive lernt that peple aint all ainjils in this wurld. their must Be sum black sheap in the flock mr. Editer, But i say and say it Boldly that no man upon God All mitys foot stule can rise an git up an say to my fase that Artemus Ward ever injered no man or woman. my new cangeroo knox the socks off from all Beasts i ever seen. its amazin to see the little Raskal holler and kick up his legs. heze a Gay one i swear to you. my wax works is the astonishment of the Elittee. yr Kolumbus Correspondant had 3 tickets to my Show charged to your offis, he said youd make it rite when i gut my hanbils struck off down to your offis. Several members of the legislater try to cum a Gouge gaim on me and kraul in to my show without Payin, but they aint Smart enough for Artemus Ward. his excellentsee guvner Chase wanted to see my Show gratooitusly, but sez i guvner all must Pay both of hi and low degre. Sez he worthy man i see the forse of yr observation and heres ten Sents. the grate man side as he saw my cangaroo. Sez he that chaned Beast remines me of the 3 milyuns an a Harf of our unfortyunate cullered brethren which air clankin their chanes down in the Slaive Ollergarchy. i make it a pint to agre with everybody which cums to my show, so i sez certinly, no dowt abowt it at all—same things o ckurred to me numerusly &c. &c. at that he shook me kordyully by the hand an sez he i wish youse wun of my constituunts. You air a hily intellijunt man. i shal go to tiffin from here. i want you to distinkly understan i shall git my hanbils dun at yr offis, but you must git up a tremendus excitement in yr Paper. you scratch my Back and ile scratch yr Back. my Snakes is as harm-lis as the new born Babe.

"'Yrs. truly. A Ward,
"'p.S—Is Haul rent hi in cleveland? Rite by next male to Tiffin. A.W.'"

"Letter from Artemus Ward—Here is another letter from Artemus Ward, proprietor of the well-known side-show:

"'Tiffin, Febey the 23th, 18&58
"'Gentz—I take my Pen in hand to inform you in regard to my kareer. Ime now in the grate Sity of tiffin. Yu better beleve the peple of tiffin

staired sum when i posted my big yeller hanbills
up in their town. No sho has bin here for going
on leven (11) years. Frequinetly the peple side
for amuzement but not a amuzement would cum.
The sity is so all fired Big that shows stan no
chanse. The hotels is all fust-class and their
bills air hyer nor showmen can ford to pay.
Howsever Artemus Ward noze no such wurd as
fale and i deturmined to storm the Mallerkarf.
if i do say it myself imes bold as a eagle. the
peple air delited with my show. my wax workd
is the prase of all. among my wax works is the
Lords last supper. the characters bein as large
as life. A feller from the east part of Seneky
County cum to my show and thot my Judus
Iscarrot was alive. Sez he to me, yo jus take
that sneakin cuss out this haul er ile smash his
hed in. Sez i young man that air is a wax work.
Sez he wax work be darned, thats ald Judus
Iscarrot and if heze a man he will step out here
and fite me. i kan stan a good deel but i gut
all fired mad, and sez i you ornary cuss keep
away from my wax works or ile fall on ye. At
that he made a lunge cross the table and seized
Judus by the neck and dragged him out inter
the middel of the haul and kommensed a poundin
him. Sez he Judus Iscarrot cant show hisself
with impunerty in tiffin by a Dam site. I
finerly convinsed the pesky fool that it was a

wax work. He larfed and said he would stan
the old rye for he and me. Tiffin is a grate city.
It is thickly settled round the meetin-house. its
princerpal institushuns air the meetin-house, hay-
scales and and William H. Gibson. mr. Gibson is on the legul tide. He tole me his bones
would be berried in Old Seneky. . . . There
was a grate competishun atween the Advertiser
and tribune to see which should strike off my
hanbils. Armstrong has got a kut of a horse
with a man holdin onto him as he said he was the
only printer in town which could do picktorial
bills, so i got my hanbills struck off up to his
offis. i shall be in Cleveland in a few weeks. i
want you should go to the gentlemunly lanlords
of the American, Weddell, Anjier, and Johnson
tavurns and git their propersishuns for keepin
me. my kompnay consists of myself two boys
a forrun Italyun who plays the hand orging, i
cangeroo, 6 snakes, calerforny bare and other
wild beasts two numerous to menshun. Set yr
hearts at rest about my Hanbills—i say they
shall be struck off down to yr offis an what i
say i mean. I shall go to toledo from tiffin.

"'yours Respectably,

Artemus Ward.

"'p.s. ive bin in the show bisness twenty-two
(22) yrs.

"'A.W.'"

"Letter from Artemus Ward—We have received another letter from Artemus Ward, proprietor of the well-known Show:

'"toledo, march 7, 18&58.
"'Gentz—For 22 yeres has the undersined bin in the show bisness and i say open and abuv bored that i was never in a more hosspital town than toledo. Awl the peple hear take a interest in my show. The haul were i exhibit is krowdid from "erly morn to dooey eve," as the Poit sez. Several of the fust famerlis of Mawmee sity and White Pidging also cum to my show. My wax works takes the peple by storm. In the langwidge of the Toledo Blaid, "Artemus Ward's wax works air chief de overs of Skulptorialastic art." Toledo is a interestin sity. There is probly more promersing and virtuous young men in toledo than there is anywheres. The climit is such that a great many of the mail inhabitants hav to take a gin-cocktale evry mornin afore brekfust. It was hard for them to do it at fust but thay take to it quite nateral now. My cangeroo gut out of his cage the other evenin and run off faster nor a lokomotive. The Common Counsil was in session at the time my cangeroo gut out and when thay heerd of the affectin casyualty they unainimersly parsed the

follering preambel and resolushuns: " ' "Whereas,
This ere Counsil thinks hily of Artemus Ward;
and Whereas, it has pleased Devine Providence
to cause his cangeroo to escaip; and Whereas,
the resunt escaip of a hyeny in Pauldin county
and his terriable doins in a grave yard planely
shows the awfulness of allowin beasts of pray to
roam through the country—therefore be it

" ' "Resolved, That this Counsil do immediately
ajurn and assist Mr. Ward for to capter his
beast."

" 'Accordingly thay did so. Abowt seving
hundred (700) citizuns jined in the pursoot. We
chased the little cuss clear up to Tremendusville
afore we cawt him. It would have made you
larf to hearn the little cuss squeal and kick up
his legs. On our return to toledo abel and
eloqunt speaches was maid by several disting-
wished citizuns, and awl parsed off in the most
pleasant stile.

" 'My snakes is under perfect subjecshun.
Among my snakes is a Boy Constructor, the
largist in the wurld. It wood make your blud
freeze to see the mongster unkoil hisself. If
yu put this letter in the paper i wish you wood
be more particlar abowt the spellin and punc-
tooation. i dont ploom myself on my learnin.
i shall be in Cleveland befour long and my han-

bills shall certinly be struck off down to your offis. Set your harts at rest on that pint.

      " 'Very Respectively yours,

                Artemus Ward.' "

His work on *The Plain Dealer* consisted of picking up any city news from the police and court items, answering mythical correspondents, as well as joking the citizens and recording the showman's adventures. As years went on his salary increased a little, but not enough, and when, in 1860, an offer came from *Vanity Fair* to duplicate his copy in their pages, the first journal to syndicate humor, he resigned his position with *The Plain Dealer*.

Ward (as he was known) did not go directly to New York, but became advance agent and business associate with Ossian E. Dodge, a singer of comic songs, then touring across Ohio, Indiana and Illinois. Dodge had the reputation of being rather "close" and his advance agent was not kept well supplied with funds. The road tour ended in Chicago and Ward went on to Pittsburgh. There he fell in with Sanford's Minstrels, and he put on burnt cork and became end-man for a few days, to the delight of Pittsburgh audiences.

He arrived in New York, January, 1861. He

refused the rival papers' offers to publish an Artemus Ward column each week in order to work on *Vanity Fair*. At the outbreak of the Civil War, Leland, the editor of *Vanity Fair* resigned, as he was not in favor of the policy the owners of the magazine proposed to follow in regard to political affairs. Artemus Ward was given his position. During the war *Vanity Fair* had a hard struggle, for the people were in no mood for a comic paper. Ward made contributions to the columns occasionally but the routine work grew irksome and the wanderlust again seized him. In the middle of the summer he travelled West as far as Louisville, where he met Dr. Hingston who later became his agent and manager.

In a month he was on the job again, though his heart was not in it. He had no head for finances and *Vanity Fair* badly needed one. He became possessed with the idea of giving a "show," since he saw no future for himself in the paper, and he began the preparation of a "piece." This was a lecture made up of a collection of old jokes from *The Plain Dealer's* local column, stories picked up about town and any nonsense which came into his mind. His first appearance was made at New London, Connecticut, on November 26, 1861. The local 'press commented so favorably upon the venture that thereafter he had no trouble in securing dates for his lectures. He traveled over New England and New York, in the next two months, and while he met with great success he had only a small income. He had no management and apparently he had no fixed sum for his lecture. He went West that spring as far as Milwaukee, concluding his tour in Cleveland, where he was warmly welcomed by his old friends.

In February, while in Maine, he met Charles Shaw, who now undertook the management of his show and contributed considerably to its financial success. In May, 1862, "Artemus Ward—His Book" was published and forty thousand copies were sold in a very short time. This was an enormous edition for that period, and the royalties brought Ward six thousand dollars. All lecture platforms were open to him now and his engagements were as many as he could comfortably fill. Shaw, though a good manager, had other interests to attend to. Ward felt the need of someone who could give him his entire time and attention, so he formed a partnership with Hingston.

He planned to write another book, but the lecture platform absorbed all his time and energy. Success stayed with him and life was easy, except when he overworked—as quite frequently he did. In October, 1863, he sailed from New York to California, via the Isthmus of Panama. His first lecture was given in San Francisco on the thirteenth of November, and was a "triumph which could seldom if ever be repeated." The hall was crowded to the doors, and as many more clamored to hear him outside.

Very much against Hingston's advice, Ward insisted upon making the return trip by land. There were no railroads that far west, so they travelled by coach and horseback. At Virginia City, Nevada, where he stopped to lecture, he made the acquaintance of Samuel L. Clemens (Mark Twain), whom he promised to help in the publication of his articles in the New York papers. When the world had its first laugh with Mark Twain, in 1865, it was due to Artemus Ward.

While in Salt Lake City, Ward was taken so sick with mountain fever that he was not expected to recover. He received tender and careful nursing, and Brigham Young himself inquired about him daily. On February 8, he was well enough to deliver his postponed lecture which was well received in Salt Lake City. He made a quick lecture tour all across the continent. From these experiences Ward wrote his lectures on the Mormons—"Their Religion was singular, but their wives were plural." Upon his return to New York, despite the heavy expenses of the trip, he deposited fifteen thousand dollars in the bank.

Ward now began to plan a new lecture to be illustrated by the Panorama which was so popular at that time. The next two seasons were very successful and included tours from Montreal to New Orleans. Upon his return from his southern trip he was quite worn out and spent several months in Waterford resting and planning for a visit to England.

He sailed from New York on June 2, 1866, and landed in England ten days later. Proceeding to London he found a warm welcome, and the summer was spent in resting and making friends. He was made a member of the famous Savage Club in August. The life he led in England soon began to show ill effects, not merely because of the strenuous entertainment in his honor, but because of the mental strain due to the continual demand to provide amusement for an expectant company. His friends noticed that he was failing, and urged him to take better care of himself and live more quietly.

The comic papers in London sought after Ward, and *Punch* secured him as a contributor. Ward regarded it "as quite the proudest moment of his life to have written for the oldest comic journal in the English language and to have been as well appreciated here as at home." His first lecture in London, given November 13, 1866, has been described as follows:

"The opening night of the show Hingston introduced him in a neat little speech and claimed the indulgence of those present for any nervousness the entertainer might display on this, his first public appearance in London. He said it was a critical moment for Ward, and his fate trembled in the balance. Then Ward rose, came down to the footlights and stood silent, casting his deep-set, brilliant eyes over the vast audience and twiddling his thumbs in the most unconcerned way. A minute or two passed; under such circumstances it seemed much longer. The audience became fidgety. I heard one gentleman sitting near me exclaim to a lady at his side: 'What a fool! Why doesn't he say something?' Once more a silence fell upon the assembly, but the imperturbable man stood twiddling his thumbs. A murmur of disapproval swept like a wave over the audience, then a little more clapping, a little more stamping, followed by a silence during which a pin might almost have been heard to fall. At last, in his inimitable drawl, Ward spoke:

"'Ladies- and- Gentlemen: When- you- have-

finished-this-unseemly-interruption, I guess I'll
begin my discourse.'

"It was as if an electric shock had passed
through the people. They saw the humor of the
situation. They rose to it. And seldom has a
showman received such an ovation. The audience almost raised the roof with its cheers of
applause, and it was fully five minutes before
he could proceed. From that moment he became
the idol of London."

For the following six weeks Ward lectured in
London, but on the seventh of January he had
become so weak that he was unable to appear
for two evenings. On January 23rd, he gave
his last lecture. He went to the island of Jersey, because the climatic conditions were considered more favorable than in London. Conditions were not what he had hoped, so he
stayed in Jersey only a short time.

At Southampton he stopped at a hotel. He
was extremely weak; as one has said of him,
"The Candle had burned too long at both ends."
Nothing could be done to save him although he
was surrounded by many and famous friends.
He had had tuberculosis, although apparently
latent, for a long time. Now the disease was in
a far advanced and hopeless stage. The nurse
had considerable difficulty in convincing him

that he should take the medicine that had been prescribed. His friend, Tom Robertson, was with him all the time and on one occasion, as Robertson attempted to give him a dose of extremely bitter iron tonic, he wittily met the arguments as follows:

"My dear Tom," said Artemus protestingly, "I can't take that dreadful stuff."

"Come, come," said Robertson, "Take it, my dear fellow, just for my sake. You know I would do anything for you."

"Would you?" said Artemus, faintly, grasping Tom's hand.

"I would indeed."

"Then you take it."

As he grew weaker and weaker, he called one day for a pencil and paper and began to jot down some biographical facts. He wrote only a few lines, however, when he was too weak to continue. He never tried to write again. He died on the afternoon of March 6, 1867. It has been said that "Never was an American in London so beloved." This was evidenced by the mourning throughout England when his death was announced. The following poem was written by James Rhoades and appeared in *The Spectator* only ten days after Ward's death.

FIGHTERS OF FATE

ARTEMUS WARD

Is he gone to a land of no laughter,
  This man who made mirth for us all?
Proves death but a silence hereafter
  From the sounds that delight or appal?
Once closed, have the lips no more duty,
  No more pleasure the exquisite ears,
Has the heart done o'erflowing with beauty
  As the eyes have with tears?

Nay, if aught be sure, what can be surer
  Than that Earth's good decays not with Earth?
And of all the heart's springs none are purer
  Than the springs of the fountains of Mirth?
He that sounds them has pierced the heart's hollows,
  The places where tears are and sleep;
For the foam-flakes that dance in life's shallows
  Are wrung from life's deep.

He came with a heart full of gladness.
  From the glad-hearted world of the West—
Won our laughter, but not with mere madness,
  Spake and joked with us, not in mere jest;
For the Man in our heart lingered after,
  When the merriment died from our ears,
And those that are loudest in laughter
  Are silent in tears.

Of Ward, Mr. Conway, of the Unitarian
Church, said: "I was requested by a committee
of Americans to conduct the funeral. . . .
and never had a more difficult or sorrowful task.
For his unexpected death was a tragedy that
almost unnerved me. The chapel in Kensal

Green Cemetery was filled to its utmost capacity. All the chief actors and actresses, writers of plays, literary men and women, were present, and sorrow was on every face." Mr. Conway said that Ward had never met with one whom he had not made his friend and had never lost a friend that he had once made. He said, too, that Ward had never made an enemy, and that there was no man who did not feel that he was better for having known him.

REFERENCES

Artemus Ward. By Don C. Seitz.
Artemus Ward. Stories of Authors. By Edwin Watts Chubb.
Artemus Ward. His Book.

SIDNEY LANIER

SIDNEY LANIER was born, February 3, 1842, in Macon, Georgia. His father was a lawyer, not any too prosperous, whose remote ancestors could be traced to the time of Queen Elizabeth. His mother was Mary Anderson from the prominent Virginia family of that name. Sidney grew up in an environment of culture, refinement and the hospitality characteristic of the old South. The value of his simple home life cannot be overestimated in its effect on his later life and writings. In early childhood he took great interest in, and showed a remarkable talent for music. His ancestry includes court musicians in the time of Elizabeth, James I and Charles I. His mother taught Sidney to read music and without further instruction he played the piano, organ, guitar, flute and violin. As a child he organized musical bands among his playmates. Later in life, he said: "The prime inclination—that is, natural bent (which I have checked, though) of my nature is to music, and for that I have the greatest talent; indeed, not boasting, for God gave it to me, I have an extraordinary musical talent and feel it within me plainly that I could rise as high as any composer."

Early in life he also showed great interest in books, cultivated in his father's library where he had the opportunity of access to the best literature. When he was sixteen years old, he entered Oglethorpe University as a sophomore. He was an excellent student and graduated, in 1860, the first in his class. He was offered a position as tutor in his Alma Mater. He took up the work gladly but leaned all the while toward a career in music and musical composition.

When the Civil War broke out, Lanier was among the first to enlist. Although he had a great dislike of war, he was promoted in the service from time to time, and throughout the entire period of the conflict he did his duty to the best of his ability. He was captured and imprisoned at Point Lookout, where he endured the hardships of prison life with a cheerfulness and bravery which won him the unending admiration of his companions. During his confinement in prison, Lanier perfected his technique of the flute, in the mastery of which he was unexcelled. His prison experience is also responsible for the break-down of his health.

The next four years were very trying for all Southern men, but Lanier never felt any bitter-

ness toward the North or resented the inevitable.
He deplored the horrors of war, in his only novel,
"Tiger Lilies," published in 1867, but his attitude
is best expressed in an address over the Con-
federate dead, given in his own home. He closed
with these words: "Today we are here for love,
and not for hate. Today we are here for harmony, and not for discord. Today we are risen
immeasurably above all vengeance. Today,
standing upon the serene heights of forgiveness,
our souls choir together the enchanting music of
harmonious Christian civilization."

In this spirit, when the war was over, he began
the struggle for existence. The war had handicapped him terribly, since along with his camp
life and his terrible experiences in prison he had
developed tuberculosis. Quite frequently he had
hemorrhages and, from time to time, he gave
up his position thinking that climatic change
would benefit his health. Immediately after
the war he accepted a position which required
the teaching of thirty classes a day on a plantation near Macon. This work proved too heavy
and he went to Mobile, Alabama, to spend the
winter, hoping to benefit his health. Following
this, he tried work as a hotel clerk at Montgomery,
Alabama, where he wrote a novel. In the spring
of 1867, Lanier went to New York to find a

publisher for his book. He then began teaching
in a small school in Prattville, Alabama. Although he was suffering from hemorrhages he
continued writing and studying.

In 1867, he married Miss Mary Day and their
marriage was nothing short of ideal. He writes
of his wife in one of his poems:

> Dear eyes, dear eyes and rare complete—
> Being heavenly-sweet and earthly-sweet—
> I marvel that God made you mine,
> For when He frowns, 'tis then ye shine!

Faced with the necessity of supporting a wife
and child, he took up the study of law and, in
1870, began to practice with his father. He was
a careful, intelligent attorney. Much as he
longed to write, he felt the necessity of provid-
ing a more substantial living than the uncertain
market for his poems would offer. Tuberculosis
continued to grip him, but he made a valiant
struggle and was always cheerful and hopeful.

At different periods in his life Lanier lived in
Texas, Florida, and North Carolina in attempts
to discover a salubrious climate. Having resolved to devote his life to music and poetry he
went to Baltimore in 1873, where he found many
friends and a means of support as first flutist in
the Peabody Orchestra. His father urged him to

return to Macon and to the practice of law; but he replied that he had had a longing to devote himself to poetry and music all his life and he must indulge it. In Baltimore were opportunities, not only to support his family by means of work dear to his heart, but also for study along the lines he had chosen.

The Johns Hopkins University was then in its infancy and Lanier became an ardent student. While there he undertook an extended course of study and reading. He made himself familiar with the works of Langland and Chaucer. He was convinced that in order to become a great poet he must possess wide knowledge. The next eight years are said to have been the happiest of his life. Under the encouragement and inspiration afforded by his family, these years became productive of great accomplishment. Despite the fact that he was weak and frequently in pain he indulged to the fullest extent his passion for music, and wrote his finest poetry. In 1879, he was appointed lecturer on English literature at Johns Hopkins University. The themes of his lectures were brought together in book form under the titles of "The Science of English Verse" and "The English Novel." He wrote several other volumes, among them "Florida," "The Boy's King. Arthur," "The

Boy's Froissart," "The Boy Percy."   During all
this time he suffered greatly, as evidenced by a
letter written to his friend Hayne, in 1880: "I
could never tell you," he says, "the extremity of
illness, of poverty, and of unceasing toil, in which
I have spent the last three years; and you would
need only once to see the weariness with which
I crawl to bed after a long day's work, and after
a long night's work at the heels of it,—and
Sundays just as well as other days,—in order to
find in your heart a full warrant for my silence.
It seems incredible that I have printed such an
unchristian quantity of matter,—all, too, toler-
ably successful,—and secured so little money;
and the wife and the four boys, who are so lovely
that I would not think a palace good enough for
them, if I had it, make one's earnings seem all
the less."

When he delivered the last of his series of
lectures, in the winter of 1880, he was so weak
that he was unable to stand to deliver them.   He
made a trip to New York to see about the publication of his existing works, and then went to
Asheville, North Carolina, believing that the
altitude and clear air might effect a partial recovery.   Later he went to Lynn, and although his
father, brother and wife, who were ever present,
knew the end was not far distant, he continually

made plans for his return to the University in the fall. He fought a desperate fight throughout the summer but, on September 7, 1881, the end came, even as he wished it might, before an open window just at sunset.

Shortly after his death, memorial services were held at Johns Hopkins University at which many beautiful tributes were paid to him by his colleagues and friends. He was buried in Baltimore and although his grave was not even marked by a slab it attracts as much interest of visitors as does the grave of Poe in the same city.

Of Lanier it has been said: "In Sidney Lanier we have a knight-errant in the cause of beauty and truth and holiness. No mail-clad warrior, out of shining fields of old romance, ever quested for fairer adventures than did this knight of our new days. And the revelation of his high and unbending nobility is to be sought not merely in his messages in prose and verse; its steady and winsome radiance is equally revealed in the very character of the man as he opened himself in frank unreservedness to all with whom he came in contact on the common way of life. So his finest poetry and its deepest spiritual message may not be read so much in rhythmic verse, as in his brave and inspiringly victorious struggle against the untoward conditions of time and circumstance, in the stubborn cheerful manliness of his combat with disease, and in an unwavering fidelity to high artistic and spiritual ideals. . . . With him there is no divorce between the man and his works; as one listens to the clear moral purity of his poetry, there is no need of a blinking apology for any soil of sin or wanderings in dark and forbidden ways on the part of the man."

REFERENCES

Sidney Lanier. American Men of Letters. By Edwin Mims.
Poets of the South. By F. V. N. Painter.
Letters of Sidney Lanier. Charles Scribner's Sons.
Sidney Lanier. Stories of Authors. By Edwin Watts Chubb.

EDWARD LIVINGSTON
TRUDEAU

EDWARD LIVINGSTON TRUDEAU was born in New York City, on October 5, 1848, of French parentage. His mother was Cephise Berger, only daughter of Dr. Francois Berger, a Parisian practicing medicine in New York, and his father was Dr. James Trudeau, a member of a well-known New Orleans family. His father and mother separated shortly after his birth. His mother and grandparents went abroad with Trudeau and his older brother, whom he adored. He received his preparatory education in Paris. When he was eighteen he returned with his grandparents to New York. This was at the close of the Civil War. For a time he attended the Columbia School of Mines and then decided to enter the United States Navy. He was admitted in a preparatory school at Newport and was about to enter the Academy when an unexpected event changed the whole course of his life.

His brother had been delicate from childhood, as a result of congenital heart trouble. Trudeau had always helped and cared for him and, consequently, they were closer than most brothers are. Trudeau, upon learning that his brother had consumption, gave up his appointment and returned to New York to care for him until he died, in December, 1865. Trudeau occupied the same room and sometimes even the same bed with his brother, for he stayed with him day and night. At that time fresh air was supposed to be most harmful, so the windows were never opened and it was not strange that, before the end came, Trudeau began to break under the strain. The physician in charge did not tell him of his great danger from contact exposure. In fact the tubercle bacillus had not yet been discovered.

For a time he was stunned by the loss of his brother and unable to settle down to any work. Later in life, he says: "It was my first great sorrow. It nearly broke my heart and I have never ceased to feel its influence." Inspired to do something that might alleviate such suffering as his brother had endured, he decided to study medicine. In the fall of 1868, he entered the College of Physicians and Surgeons of New York. The year before his graduation he became engaged to Miss Charlotte Beare, of Little Neck, Long Island, and having subsequently served a six months interneship at the Stranger's Hospital, they were married in June, 1871. They sailed for Europe at once, returning in October. Dr. Trudeau was then offered a partnership with Dr. Fessenden Otis and his future seemed very bright.

While still a medical student, he had developed a cold abscess. He consulted a physician, but the abscess did not heal until it had been operated upon several times. In those days physicians did not know that a cold abscess is often a manifestation of tuberculosis, and consequently Trudeau was not warned of his future danger. It must be borne in mind that he had previously had a long and intimate contact exposure to tuberculosis while caring for his brother. While on their honeymoon in England, Dr. Trudeau had consulted a physician because of the swelling of lymph nodes along the side of his neck. At that time this chronic condition was known as scrofula, or "The King's Evil." This was the same condition for which Samuel Johnson was touched by Queen Anne. At that time, however, no one knew that scrofula is, in reality, tuberculosis of the lymph nodes of the neck. Thus the second manifestation of tuberculosis passed with no note of warning of his impending future. Trudeau's general debility led his physician to advise the use of plenty of bacon for breakfast; to prescribe an iron tonic and had him paint the lymph nodes with iodine.

After his return to America, Dr. Trudeau had suffered occasional attacks of fever, but he attributed them to malaria, a very common disease at that time. Finally he consented, somewhat jokingly, to be examined; and it was as though sentence of death had been passed upon him when he learned that he had "tuberculosis." In those days, pulmonary tuberculosis was considered absolutely fatal. He dreaded to tell his wife, for they were very happy in their home with their first baby; but she was very brave, and together they tried to plan for the future. He had been advised to go south, so they left at once for Aiken. Here he was told to live out-of-doors and ride horseback, with the result that he developed daily fever and was no better when they returned to New York.

A week after the birth of his second child, on May 18, 1873, Dr. Trudeau accompanied by Mr. Louis Livingston, set out for Paul Smith's in the Adirondacks. The Adirondacks were chosen, not for any expected benefit of climate, but simply because Dr. Trudeau loved the forest and the wild life. Since it seemed that he had so short a time to live, he longed for surroundings he loved. It was a hard trip. After arriving at the station he had to ride forty-two miles in a wagon, over a rough corduroy road, and was almost exhausted before he was carried up to his bed. Dr. Trudeau says that as Mrs. Smith's brother placed him in the bed he had a pained expression and made the comforting remark, "Why, Doctor, you don't weigh no more than a dried lamb-skin!" The next morning when settled in a boat and rowed far down the river, where without even sitting upright he killed a deer, he began to feel better and his spirits rose. All that summer he continued to improve and the rest, good food, good general care, and open air life led to a disappearance of his symptoms. He spent entire days in a boat, fishing or being rowed about from place to place; and so was unconsciously made to rest.

In September, he returned to New York, sun-burned and fifteen pounds heavier, to rejoin his wife and babies. He was anxious to return to work, but a recurrence of certain symptoms proved to him that work would be impossible. His physician urged a winter in St. Paul, Minnesota, since it was believed that in winter Minnesota is an excellent place for persons suffering from pulmonary tuberculosis. He says: "The winter in St. Paul was not a success and, as I was allowed to drive and walk and go duck-hunting when I felt equal to it, I had some fever most of the time. By spring I was nearly as sick as the year before and the Adirondacks seemed my only hope; so we left St. Paul in May, and early in June, accompanied by my wife, the two children, and two nurses, I arrived at Paul Smith's to my intense joy, for I always loved the place." Again his improvement was marked, and that fall he decided to try the experiment of a winter in the Adirondacks.

Contrary to the expectations of all his friends he not only survived the winter, but thrived upon it. He began to consider seriously the possible advantage, in pulmonary diseases, of exposure to pure cold air. That summer he began to practice a little among the guests at Paul Smith's the guides, and their families.

Another winter came and the Trudeau's left Paul Smith's and moved to Saranac Lake,—then only a tiny hamlet with a saw mill, a small hotel for guides, and perhaps a dozen houses. The first winters at Saranac Lake were all hunting winters, for hunting was a sport Dr. Trudeau never lost interest in and continued to enjoy even when he had to be carried in a chair from one point to another. The summers were spent at Paul Smith's where he practiced medicine.

When they returned to Saranac Lake, the

second winter, several invalids were there for
the winter, and the town had begun to grow.
Dr. Walton had regularly sent to Dr. Trudeau a
medical journal known as *The English Practitioner*. It was in 1882, while reading this
journal that Dr. Trudeau's eyes fell upon an
article giving an account of Brehmer's Sanatorium
in Silesia and of Brehmer's and Dettweiler's
epoch-making view on the treatment of tuberculosis. It was remarkable how closely the
methods they employed, coincided with those
he had independently found to be so successful
in his own practice. That winter Dr. Trudeau
dreamed his dream on the fox-run-way on the
side of Mount Pisgah, now the site of The Trudeau Sanatorium.

The idea was to build a place where patients
of moderate means could come for treatment
and where the sanatorium method could be
tried. Then began what Dr. Trudeau called
his "begging days," for since he gave his services
free of charge he felt free to ask for money for
his sanatorium. It is significant that from the
first, friends flocked to his aid, because they had
faith in him, however uncertain the work
appeared to be.

Before the Sanatorium could be started came
the wonderful year when Koch announced his

discovery of the tubercle bacillus. Trudeau was very anxious to read his discoveries in detail, but since he could not read German, he felt it would be of no use to try and obtain the article. To his delight, his friend, Mr. C. M. Lea, presented him with a hand-written copy of a full translation of Koch's famous paper. His deductions and theories were a revelation to Trudeau. All that winter, during brief visits to New York, he struggled to learn the first principles of bacteriology in order to teach himself the rest.

Trudeau was one of the first in this country to stain the tubercle bacillus, and actually bring it within range of human vision. He was firmly convinced that when tubercle bacilli were found in the sputum the patient had tuberculosis, even in the absence of all other signs and symptoms. Although he met with some difficulties he was usually able to convince others of this fact. He cites the case of a neighboring general practitioner who often visited Saranac Lake. This physician had been skeptical about germs causing tuberculosis, but asked Dr. Trudeau to convince him by examining sputum from five of his patients. The specimens arrived in five tubes, each tube numbered but without any further information. Dr. Trudeau found tubercle bacilli present in three of them. When the physician received the report he was thoroughly convinced, because the three cases in whose sputum the bacilli were found were definite cases of tuberculosis and the others were not. Another very interesting case was that of a young college graduate who, after examination, was told he had tuberculosis. He replied to Dr. Trudeau that it was impossible, since he had recently passed an examination by two of the great life insurance companies and had been insured for large sums. A little later one of these companies wrote Dr. Trudeau, asking upon what he based his diagnosis in the case of this young man. His reply was: "That the symptoms were very suspicious, but that the presence of the bacillus, to my mind, was irrefutable evidence of the presence of a tuberculous process as their cause." This finding so convinced the insurance company that one of its physicians was sent to Dr. Trudeau to learn the new method of diagnosing tuberculosis.

Dr. Trudeau's meager laboratory facilities were the beginning of the laboratory study of tuberculosis in the United States. This laboratory was a little room in the wing of his house heated only by a wood-stove, where he struggled with a home-made thermostat, heated by a kerosene lamp, until he succeeded in grow-

ing the tubercle bacillus outside of the human
body. The guinea-pigs used for repeating all
Koch's experiments he had to keep in a hole
underground, heated by a kerosene lamp. One
of his first experiments proved that rabbits, inoculated with the disease and then turned loose on
an island and well-fed, recovered in the fresh air;
while others, similarly inoculated and kept in
unhygienic places, died in a very short time.
Thus began the first experimental work in tuberculosis in the United States. Little did Trudeau
know that in less than one-half century the
experimental work which he began would be
carried on in many centers of the country and
would seriously threaten the strongholds of the
tubercle bacillus.

Dr. Trudeau's description of how the first
patients were admitted to the sanatorium and
the treatment they received, follows: "The building of a little rough-board barn and a portion of
the main building had progressed sufficiently,
by the middle of the summer of 1884, to enable
Mr. Norton to move his family in and live on the
place. Late in the fall Dr. Loomis sent up the
first two patients,—two sisters, both factory
girls; one Alice Hunt, had pulmonary tuberculosis; and the other, Mary Hunt, had had Pott's
disease and now showed slight evidences of

pulmonary tuberculosis as well. Dr. Loomis had found someone willing to pay their expenses and had sent them up on this account, as nothing would have been done for them at their home, a crowded tenement. They were both in wretched health, poorly clad to stand the Adirondack winter cold, and were nearly dead with fatigue when they reached the Sanatorium, after a forty-two-mile drive from Ausable Forks. Mrs. Norton and her daughters took them right into the family circle; my wife got some warm clothes for them; and I examined them and advised them as to what to do, and encouraged them to the best of my ability.

At that time only the foundations and frame of the first little cottage had been built; and the cottage was not completed and occupied until February 1, 1885. In looking at it now it seems rather curious why it should have been delayed so long, for it certainly was a most modest undertaking; but with neither men nor money available, I imagine Mr. Riddle did all that could be done under the circumstances. This first cottage consisted of one room, fourteen by eighteen, and a little porch so small that only one patient could sit out at a time, and with difficulty. It was furnished with a wood-stove, two cot-beds, a wash-stand, two chairs and a kerosene lamp, and cost, as I remember, about four hundred dollars when completed. The money was obtained by Mr. C. M. Lea from a Mrs. Jenks, a lady in Philadelphia.

This humble little building has become somewhat historical now, and has always been known at the Sanatorium as "The Little Red." Humble as it undoubtedly is, it was nevertheless the pioneer cottage in the development of the sanatorium treatment in America, and has stood for a great principle of treatment which will long survive the little building. At present it is kept in repair as a relic, and used as a little museum for other relics connected with the history of the institution."

The Sanatorium continued to grow, though slowly. The main building was finished in 1886 and two more cottages were added; but there was no coal and no running water. Dr. Trudeau was full of hope, but he had no definite ideas of what to do and very little money with which to do anything. He could not afford a resident physician and had to do the medical work himself, driving in summer fourteen miles from Paul Smith's at each visit.

There were no nurses, nor any one to direct the patients or attend to them. In fact there were many dark days for the little sanatorium, but, in 1888, things began to grow better. Mrs. Julia Miller became Superintendent and Mr. Frank Ingersoll, a medical student who was also a patient, was able to assist Dr. Trudeau materially in the medical work. That same year the first fair was held at Saranac Inn and since that time fairs have been held there and at Paul Smith's regularly. This is one of the main sources of support for the work of the institution.

As Saranac Lake became better known through Dr. Trudeau's efforts, many loyal friends, out of gratitude for what he had done for them, as well as for the world in general, made generous contributions,—with the result that the Adirondack Cottage Sanatorium became one of the best equipped of its kind in the country. Where once stood but a single cottage, the institution now covers many acres, with everything from a nurses' training school to a modern, well-equipped laundry.

In 1877, the second son, Henry, was born, and in 1887, Francis, a third son was born. The first great sorrow that Dr. and Mrs. Trudeau together shared was the death of the second baby boy, who developed convulsions and died three days later. The children always received excellent care and training. Writing of the older children, Dr. Trudeau says: "Chatte was

a strong, athletic girl, with a vigorous body and
eyes as black as coal. She was very fond of
rowing, tennis, riding horse-back and all violent
exercises, and had never shown any sign of illness. Ned was slighter, but very wiry and
active." In the fall of 1887, Dr. and Mrs.
Trudeau sent Chatte to a girl's school in
New York. From the letters she wrote home
at first it was evident that she was quite home-
sick. Soon after Christmas she wrote that she
was not feeling well. There seemed to be no
improvement in her health as time passed, so
Dr. Trudeau asked her to come home for the
Easter vacation. She returned and Dr. Trudeau's own description of her appearance and
its stunning effect upon him and her mother
follows: "I met her at the train and brought her
home, and I never shall forget the shock her
appearance gave me. From a plump, robust
young woman she had changed to a pale, listless
girl, and as she went upstairs to see her mother
I went into my office and shut the door. The
terrible truth flashed upon me as I remembered
how my brother appeared when he was taken ill
and came to see me in Newport. I knew it was
the same old story, and I felt stunned and had
to wait a long time to get hold of myself again
before joining the family circle. I at once made

up my mind I must know the truth, and alarm her as little as possible. It was my responsibility and I could share it with no one, so I did a piece of acting that day which I shall never forget, with a smile on my face and a breaking heart; for before night I knew the truth in all its shocking details, and yet no one in the school, none of our friends who saw her constantly, had suspected it! I told my wife at once. I have always told her everything, and we have always borne together whatever we have had to bear. As usual, in spite of the terrible shock, she was calm and hopeful. For some mysterious reason I was much less so. I felt from the first this was the same type of disease my brother had; the type that progresses rapidly and against which treatment is of no avail."

In speaking of Dr. Trudeau's diagnosis in Chatte's case, Dr. Allen K. Krause says: "On rare occasions he used to speak about it. Her appearance when she stepped from the train, frightened him; to his trained eye her look was that of a consumptive, with fearful and heavy heart he drove her home. It was early in the evening, and as the family sat down to dinner, he went up to Chatte's room to look for her handkerchief. He found this, took it into his laboratory at the earliest possible moment, removed a particle of material from it, made a smear of this, stained the smear and found the bacilli, tubercle bacilli."

During the next few years, although apparently better at times, she fought a losing battle and toward the last she suffered a great deal. Her death, in March, 1893, was a terrible blow to her parents.

While Chatte was ill, Ned had gone to Yale where he not only proved himself an excellent student but also an athlete. He was made pitcher of the freshman baseball team. Later he was made pitcher on the university team and "pitched Yale to victory in some of the great intercollegiate matches." In 1900, he graduated at the College of Physicians and Surgeons, having been elected to the presidency of his class. After serving an interneship he returned to Saranac Lake to help his father. Here again, Dr. Trudeau manifested his wonderful spirit by making a tremendous sacrifice for the sake of his son Ned. Much as he cared for him and much as he needed his assistance, Dr. Trudeau felt that it was not best for Ned to locate permanently in Saranac Lake, because he says, "I was beginning already to realize the stigma with which the world stamps everything and everybody connected with tuberculosis."

Ned married Miss Hazel Martyn of Chicago; and the young couple located in New York City, where Ned began his practice with Dr. James of that city. Dr. Trudeau says that when he saw Ned with such wonderful opportunities "I rejoiced then I had not let him assume a more obscure career with his father in the remote little Adirondack village, with its ever-present burden of chronic illness." In the spring of this same year Dr. James wired Dr. Trudeau that "Ned had been suddenly taken down with an acute pneumonia." The parents rushed to Ned's bedside to find him very ill. However, the crisis passed and it seemed certain he would recover. The termination is best told by Dr. Allen K. Krause: "Ned had successfully weathered the crisis of his disease and was on the way back to health. Everyone was in high feather; so, one afternoon, the doctor left Mrs. Trudeau with a happy party at his host's home and went to visit Ned at the hospital, to make arrangements to take him home the next week, where he might complete his convalescence. He found Ned sitting up, mending rapidly and in such good condition that he was to be discharged from the hospital within a few days; and after a happy hour with his son he left, to join the party at tea and carry the good news to Mrs. Trudeau."

The Doctor would then tell this story:

"He opened the front door of the house. As he stepped inside he heard the laughter and animated talk of the company upstairs. The butler rushed up to him and told him that the hospital had just called him by telephone. He went to the telephone and from the other end of the wire the hospital resident called to him: 'My God, Doctor, I believe Ned's dead.' He sensed the truth at once, pulmonary embolism. Crushed and dazed he dropped the receiver. He made his way to the stairs and clung to the post. From above came the sounds of light-hearted gaiety, but within a minute or two his resolution was made. As best he could, up the stairs, across the hall, to the door of the room, he made his way. The party greeted him loudly and cheerily, but he had but one thought—he wanted to see 'Lottie' outside, in the hall.

"When his wife came he looked at her. 'I'd have rather struck her a blow between the eyes with a sledge. But, as I looked at her,—as she looked at me,—I saw that she could stand it, and I told her the truth,'—he would say simply."

The only remaining child, Francis B., was a great comfort to his parents as old age crept upon them. He became a physician and now practices in Saranac Lake.

Among the patients at Saranac Lake was Robert Louis Stevenson and many were the pleasant evenings that Dr. Trudeau and Stevenson spent before the fire in the winter of 1887. It was during that winter, while he was under Dr. Trudeau's care, that Stevenson produced many of his greatest essays.

During the last years of his life, Dr. Trudeau was confined much to his bed, but his work went steadily forward in the hands of his able assistants. He lived to see the celebration of the twenty-fifth anniversary of the Sanatorium's existence, on February 15, 1910, when he was presented with a beautiful book containing over one thousand congratulatory cards from former patients who had recovered their health at the Sanatorium.

Artificial pneumothorax treatment was being recommended in certain parts of the world and, approximately two years before his death, Dr. Trudeau had this administered. He had studied this method of treatment carefully and it is now said, by those who knew him best, that he wanted this treatment administered in his own case, more to express his firm faith in it and to encourage others whose years might be greatly extended by its use, than for any benefit which he himself might derive from it. Another manifestation of his wonderful spirit!

There is nothing that a professional man enjoys more than the confidence and respect of the members of his own profession. No American physician had more enjoyment from this source than Dr. Trudeau. Such great leaders in the medical profession, as Dr. Osler (Sir William), Dr. Janeway, Dr. Loomis, Dr. Linsley Williams, Dr. Allen K. Krause, Dr. Lawrason Brown, Dr. E. B. Baldwin, Dr. Hermann M. Biggs, Dr. James Alexander Miller, Dr. Walter B. James and many others manifested the greatest confidence in him; they did all in their power to aid him and support his work, and were ever ready to comfort and encourage him in times of sorrow and disappointment. In addition to these outstanding individuals, great medical societies bestowed upon him the highest honors within their power. Having been elected to Membership in the American Climatological Association, Dr. Trudeau was invited to read a paper before the meeting, in Baltimore, in May, 1887. Although his paper was well prepared, it was Trudeau's first presentation of one before a scientific society. He started to leave just as his place on the program was reached but he fainted before he reached the door. His good friend, Dr. Loomis, read the paper for him and it brought forth much favorable com-

ment from medical men and journals both in
this country and abroad.

When the National Association for the Study
and Prevention of Tuberculosis (now known as
the National Tuberculosis Association) was
organized in 1904, Dr. Trudeau was elected as
its first president. When the International
Congress on Tuberculosis met in Washington,
in 1908, Dr. Trudeau greeted the delegates as
follows: "For thirty-five years I have lived in
the midst of a perpetual epidemic, struggling
with tuberculosis, both within and without the
walls, and no one can appreciate better than I
do the great meaning of such a meeting. I have
lived through many of the long and dark years
of ignorance, hopelessness, and apathy, when
tuberculosis levied its pitiless toll on human
life unheeded and unhindered; when, as Jaccoud
has tersely put it, 'The treatment of tuberculosis
was but a meditation on death.' But I have
lived also to see the dawn of the new knowledge,
to see the fall of the death-rate of tuberculosis,
to see hundreds who have been rescued, to see
whole communities growing up of men and
women whose lives have been saved, and who are
engaged in saving the lives of others. I have
lived to see the spread of the new light from
nation to nation until it has encircled the globe

and finds expression today in the gathering of the International Congress of Tuberculosis, with all that it means to science, philanthropy, and the brotherhood of men."

He was, later, elected President of the Congress of American Physicians and Surgeons and delivered his presidential address before this great body in Washington, in 1910. The conditions under which this was prepared have been described by A. L. Donaldson as follows: "He had been suffering from one of his most serious relapses,—high fever, acute coughing spells, and broken sleep. He awoke in the small hours of each morning, and lay tossing uncomfortably on his bed. Then it occurred to him that instead of lying there idly between coughs, thinking of himself and his troubles, he might better concentrate his mind on some preparation for the great meeting over which he had been asked to preside. So he turned on the light near his bed, reached for pad and pencil, and began the rough draft of this notable address on 'Optimism.' Not long after he was able to leave his bed and deliver it in person. What it means to turn out optimistic literature under such conditions only those who have tasted them can realize; but the unusual feat is essentially typical of Dr. Trudeau's whole career."

Moreover, honors were conferred upon him by such great educational institutions as Columbia University, McGill University and the University of Pennsylvania.

Dr. Trudeau enjoyed the respect, confidence and admiration of many outside of his own profession, evidenced by the great amount of help and encouragement he received from so prominent people as Robert Louis Stevenson, C. M. Lea, Mrs. A. J. Milbank, Samuel Inslee, George C. Cooper, Otis H. Childs, E. H. Harriman, and many others. So grateful were his former sanatorium patients that soon after his death fifteen hundred of them erected a beautiful memorial facing the view, where, as he said, "the mountains, covered with an unbroken forest, rose so abruptly from the river, and the sweep of the valley at their base was so extended and picturesque, that the view had always made a deep impression on me."

He was ever ready to help those in trouble. It is said that at one time a friend came in and told him of a poor family who had sent him to get medicine, whereupon Dr. Trudeau wrote on a prescription pad, "A sack of flour and a strip of bacon." He handed his prescription to the friend and said, "Here is some money; get that prescription filled at the store and take it to them."

The January, 1925, number of the *Journal of the Outdoor Life* was devoted to the life and work of Dr. Trudeau in commemoration of the fortieth anniversary of the Trudeau sanatorium. In this splendid number of the *Journal* are short contributions from several of Dr. Trudeau's sanatorium patients. These tributes express finely the feeling of his patients toward him and show well the value of the treatment he used in the restoration to health of the tuberculous.

Dr. Trudeau was not solely interested in the activities of his own profession. He took great interest and pride in the civic affairs of Saranac Lake. He was steadfast in his religion. He did not like to live where there was no church. He believed that a church is essential to the welfare of every community. If none existed where he lived he built one. Indeed he built three. In writing of the need he felt for church service, while at Paul Smith's he says: "During the long winter at Paul Smith's my wife and I greatly missed any opportunity to attend church services. So strong was my desire to supply this need, as far as possible, for the guides' families, that during the long winter months I used to go to the little school-house on the road to Bloomingdale and hold Sunday School for the children. I don't believe I was a very competent teacher, but it quieted my conscience to try to do something to carry the blessed message to those children who had so little opportunity to hear it."

Dr. Trudeau, in order to satisfy the longing of himself and family, set out to build a church near Paul Smith's. He appealed to his friends who came forth with money, materials and labor and the result was "St. John's in the Wilderness," which was deeded to the Board of Missions of the Episcopal Church and was consecrated in September, 1877. This church has been visited by thousands of persons and many very famous church dignitaries have held services there. It is a great inspiration to visit and attend services in it.

After moving to Saranac Lake, Dr. Trudeau was placed in charge of the building of another church which was finished early in 1879, the same year becoming the property of the Board of Missions of the Protestant Episcopal Church. This church has done and continues to do a great service to the people of Saranac Lake and like "St. John's in the Wilderness" has been visited by multitudes of people.

As the sanatorium grew, Dr. Trudeau felt that there was great need for a chapel on the grounds where the ambulant patients would have an opportunity to attend church services. In 1896, he made known his desire for a chapel on the sanatorium grounds to Mrs. Frederick Baker, who immediately made a gift of such a chapel as a memorial to her son. Because of the cosmopolitan nature of his people Dr. Trudeau thought it would be better not to have this chapel consecrated, since he desired to have it free for services to be held by clergymen of all denominations. It has indeed proved to be a wonderful institution, where the patients of the sanatorium, as well as large numbers of visitors, have profited greatly from services conducted and addresses given without price by many famous persons.

Perhaps nothing in the whole field of medicine, in the past fifty years in America, has done so much directly or indirectly to relieve suffering and extend the years of usefulness of so many people as the principle which Dr. Trudeau laid down at Saranac Lake. Only a man of unusual characteristics and an exceptionally strong personality is capable of directing an institution in such a remarkable manner.

It was Trudeau who had such a marvelous memory that he did not need to take notes on paper, and examined his patients so frequently and with such personal interest that he carried in his mind their physical conditions at all times.

It was he who wanted to help people who needed help, but asked nothing for himself.

It was he who made many scientific statements, not one of which has ever been proved to be incorrect.

It was he who did the first experimental work in tuberculosis in this country, thus making valuable contributions to our knowledge of this disease.

It was he who opened the first laboratory for the study of tuberculosis in America in which large numbers of physicians and laboratory workers have been well instructed.

It was he who was among the first to grasp the principle of tuberculosis immunity.

It was he who contributed extensively to medical literature, thus greatly extending the knowledge of physicians in the detection and treatment of tuberculosis. Probably nothing has ever been written which has served to inspire and encourage so many tuberculous patients as has his autobiography.

It was he who, among the first, stained and visualized the tubercle bacillus in this country, and then so willingly and freely instructed others.

It was he who practiced medicine, not for

financial remuneration alone—although probably few have had greater opportunities to make money—but who placed opportunities for study, discovery and service far above material reward.

It was he who through fairness, perseverance, imagination and optimism built that pioneer sanatorium which has developed a capacity of approximately 160, has treated more than 6,500 patients, and today stands in the front rank of such institutions of the world, not only from the standpoint of treatment but also from the standpoint of scientific production.

Think of this man who through all the years, accomplishing these wonderful achievements, was suffering from tuberculosis and at times experiencing the deepest of human sorrow! Truly, every tuberculous patient should take courage.

REFERENCES

Autobiography: Edward Livingston Trudeau, M.D.
A History of the National Tuberculosis Association. By S. A. Knopf.
The Beloved Physician. By Stephen Chalmers.
The Journal of the Outdoor Life, January, 1925.

CECIL JOHN RHODES

CECIL RHODES was born on July 5, 1853, the fourth of nine sons of the Rector of Bishop's Stortford, the Reverend F. W. Rhodes. His early youth was undistinguished by any remarkable brilliance or ability. A dreamy, carelessly dressed youth, fond of reading and preferring to be alone, no one would have dreamed that the future of a great continent was bound up in that life and brain. After an uneventful school career he entered Oriel College, Oxford. He was undecided as to his future vocation and thought vaguely of the ministry. The first break in his health came in 1870, when he was but sixteen years old. His lungs became affected, following a chill which developed after rowing, and he was ordered on a long sea-voyage. At that time sea-voyages were believed to be very helpful in the treatment of tuberculosis. Indeed they had been prescribed throughout the preceding 1600 years since the time when Aretaeus said: "Living on the sea will be beneficial. For the sea-water contributes something desiccant to the ulcers." The sea voyage allows a period of rest both physical and mental. It usually furnishes good food, taken at regular intervals, as well as the breathing of fresh pure air. It is these factors, rather than any drying effect upon the lungs, which bring about improvement of patients on sea-voyages.

His elder brother, Herbert, had a plantation in South Africa, and the climate of Natal induced the young man to join him. In that year, 1870, the first diamond rush to Kimberley occurred and Herbert Rhodes, tired of the slow results of farming, turned to the diamond fields. He wrote to his brother to join him; a year later Rhodes did so and the brothers worked a claim together until 1874. The claim turned out well, but Herbert was restless again and turned it over to Cecil. Herbert went further north to the more adventurous gold fields where, unfortunately, he met an untimely death. Rhodes said his brother Herbert first inspired him with the idea of acquiring the land, now known as Rhodesia, for the British Empire.

Not satisfied with the hard work in the diamond fields, Rhodes' energy found outlet in such money-making schemes as pumping out the mines and developing an ice manufacturing plant. He went back to Oxford, and only three years after his first break in health came a second illness. This time his physician gave him only six months to live. He returned at once to South Africa because he was a firm believer in the benefits of its climate and because his financial interests were developing there. His health was so well restored that, three years later (1876) he was able to return to Oxford. He spent his summer vacation in South Africa, and so maintained his recovered health that he was able to take the Bachelor of Arts and Master of Arts degrees in 1881.

The amalgamation of the diamond mines which were inefficient because of over-production and over-competition, and the formation in 1888 of the DeBeers Consolidated Mines, were the results of twenty years of effort on the part of Rhodes. The DeBeers Consolidated Mines now owns or controls all the diamond mines of any importance, thus creating a monopoly and limiting the output to supply only the world's demands. Hence, it is one of the greatest and wealthiest private concerns in the world. In this work Rhodes became associated with D. C. Rudd, who was afterwards his partner in the Rudd-Rhodes Syndicate, promoters of the British South Africa Company. When the gold fields of the Rand were discovered, in 1886, he joined with Mr. Rudd and founded the Gold Fields of South Africa. So, with unlimited wealth and

power back of him, and with a following of
moneyed men who had learned from experience
to trust him, he turned to the most gigantic
venture of all, the famous Chartered Company
of South Africa.

He made a profound study of that portion of
the continent which seemed fit for colonization
by white men and had accurate reports of its
fine climate and great fertility and of the possibilities of profitable gold fields. He knew that
to financial power must be added political power
before his dream of expansion could come true,
and with that idea in mind he went into politics.
He entered the Cape Parliament, as member for
Barkley West, and went down to the Cape
Assembly.

The details of his career in politics and the
subsequent events which led to the acquisition
of Bechuanaland and the country which now
bears his name, are too numerous to mention,
but he worked untiringly and unceasingly toward
that one end, without support or encouragement from any of the Cape Politicians. True,
the Assembly approved the plan, but it was
unwilling to undertake the expense of development and administration and, after much discouragement, Mr. Rhodes was reluctantly convinced that the only chance of carrying out his

[213]

policy lay in the creation of a private enterprise,
—a chartered company.

President Kruger, the leader of the Dutch in
South Africa, wanted the north country for his
own uses, and endeavored to block Rhodes'
route to the north by the establishment of small
Boer republics in the native territories of Bechuanaland. Rhodes, resolved to keep Bechuanaland
for England and hoping for a peaceful settle-
ment of the controversy, agreed to let the Boers
hold their farms, but only under the British
flag. This compromise was refused and there
seemed nothing to do but oust the Dutchmen;
to this end an expedition, under Sir Charles
Warren, was sent to occupy Bechuanaland.
There was some skirmishing before the expedition arrived, but a peaceful occupation was
effected; and then Rhodes renewed his offer to
give the Boers titles to the farms they had
settled. The fair-minded and generous terms,
offered by an Englishman, surprised the Boers
and probably laid the foundation of the confidence in Rhodes which enabled him to work
successfully with the Dutch of the colony.

Thus, by steadfast devotion to one idea,
Rhodes had possessed himself, by 1889, both
of financial and political power and had obtained a royal charter for the British South

Africa Company. Generally admitted to be the ablest man of affairs at the Cape, Mr. Rhodes, in 1890, became Premier of South Africa, thus combining in himself the management of the Chartered Company with the leadership of Cape Colony. An alliance with Mr. Hofmyer and the powerful Afrikander Bund secured the solid Dutch vote. Probably it was Hofmyer's intention to use Mr. Rhodes to advance his own schemes for Dutch supremacy in South Africa. If this was his plan, he had certainly reckoned without his host, for Mr. Rhodes used his position and influence so successfully that he made the occupation of Rhodesia acceptable to the Dutchmen even though it cut off the Dutch in the Transvaal from their coveted route to the north.

In 1898, Rhodes was reappointed chairman of the British South Africa Company, at a general meeting in London, and received an ovation probably greater than any ever accorded to any private individual at the British Capitol. Very much pleased and thoroughly convinced of the whole-hearted support of the shareholders, Rhodes returned to the Cape and threw himself with all his energy into the development of the north.

Mr. Rhodes, as all rich men are, was constantly

besieged with requests for financial assistance from all parts of the world. As a rule, he lent a ready ear to such applicants and it has been estimated that he gave away money at the rate of a hundred pounds (£ 100) a day. He was generous to a fault and, always preferring to use his own judgment, he often gave to those whom he had been told were totally undeserving. Outwardly, he appeared to have a rather gruff and forbidding manner, but anyone who knew him well knew that the real man was the Cecil Rhodes who wrote, "I am so sorry for all your troubles." That was the keynote of his feeling toward all his fellow creatures, white or black, rich or poor. His religion can be summed up in his own words: "An effort for the betterment of one's fellow beings," and he practised it in the alleviation of suffering and want wherever he went.

The absolute, unquestioning confidence which Rhodes placed in all men whom he selected to aid him in this work made them unhesitatingly follow him with blind trust, secure in the knowledge that "Rhodes would see everything put right." Some mention should be made of the great friendship between Rhodes and Dr. Jameson, who figured so prominently in the Jameson Raid. Dr. Jameson was looked upon as a foremost figure in his profession in Africa and he had an enormous practice. He disliked politics exceedingly, but his loyalty to Rhodes induced him to enter the ring. He attended Rhodes constantly in his last illness; and after his death the same loyalty to his friend kept Jameson interested in affairs, despite the fact that it was work he detested.

Toward the end of 1901, Rhodes' health declined rapidly and he returned home where he began negotiating for the purchase of Dalham Hall, Newmarket, where he hoped to prolong his life in the cooler climate of England. An unexpected event taxed his strength and he became weaker and weaker, until it was clear that no hope remained. Toward the end he felt a strong desire to return to England. Despite the fact that he was told that he could not live to reach the dock, he clung to the idea and cabins were reserved and fitted out with electric fans and oxygen tanks in readiness for him. But, on the day he was to have sailed, the end came. Conscious to the last, he died with the words, "So little done, so much to do," on his lips.

His body lay in state for two days at "Groote Shuur," and it was estimated that at least thirty-five thousand people passed through the house. It was then taken under an escort of

Cape police to the House of Parliament for a second lying-in-state. From there the body went by special train to Bulawayo and at every station, through which the train passed, there was a guard of honor drawn up and crowds of people of every nationality waiting to pay their last tribute. On April 10, 1902, the body was finally laid to rest on the hill, that Rhodes himself had selected as the site for his grave, which he called "The World's View."

In his will, Rhodes made sufficient provision for his family, but the bulk of his wealth went into scholarships for his beloved Oxford. It has been said that America has, in proportion to those allotted to the British Empire, too large a percentage of these scholarships. However, Rhodes felt the tie of language to be a very strong one and hoped to lay a foundation for a closer union between the Mother country and all the great Anglo-Saxon races by means of the same educational tie. It is of interest to note, in passing, that McDugald McLean, from Texas, who later suffered and died of tuberculosis, was granted one of these scholarships. Rhodes added a codicil allotting five scholarships to German students, to the end that an understanding might be brought about between these three great Powers of the world by means of the strongest tie that he could conceive, that of educational relations, hoping that the existence of such understanding might ensure the peace of the world; in fact, as he hoped, make war impossible.

REFERENCES

Cecil Rhodes: The Man and His Work. By Gordon LeSueur.
Cecil Rhodes: Empire Builder. By John Tombs. *The Journal of the Outdoor Life*, May, 1923.
Cecil Rhodes: A Biography and Appreciation. By Imperialist and Dr. Jameson.

CHRISTOPHER MATHEWSON

CHRISTOPHER MATHEWSON was born in Factoryville, Pennsylvania, on August 12, 1880. His parents were of Puritan stock. As a boy Christopher was very proficient in curving flat stones. At the age of twelve years he announced to his mother his ambition to become a baseball pitcher. This announcement had been foreshadowed a year earlier by his earning enough money to purchase for himself a good baseball.

Factoryville, then a small town of about 800 inhabitants, had a baseball team composed of grown men. When Christopher was only fourteen years old, the local baseball team was without a pitcher. Some one who had seen Christopher pitch suggested that the boy be given a chance, despite his age. Proving his mettle at the forenoon practice, Christopher was chosen to pitch the regular game that afternoon, although it was not on the home field. Christopher did pitch and Factoryville won. This was the beginning of his popularity as a pitcher in his home community. From that time on he was frequently called upon to pitch for a local academy team and for the Factoryville team.

Then he was offered a dollar a game to pitch for a neighboring town team. Here he earned his first money as a baseball pitcher, although he had to walk five miles to the town and five miles back after the game was over. Later, he went to Bucknell College and his popularity as a baseball player followed him. There he played not only baseball, but football. During summer vacations he earned small sums of money and, later, as much as twenty to eighty dollars a month by playing baseball with the Hinesdale and the Norfolk teams in the Virginia league. In fact, it was through the Norfolk team that he went to New York in 1900.

His experience at the tryout is described by Cary, as follows: "The manager himself—not John McGraw, but his predecessor—took the bat.

" 'Now,' he said, 'Let's see what you got.'

" 'Christy gave him his first ball. The manager struck but missed. He shook his head admiringly.

" 'Your fast one is all right,' he said, 'How about your curve?'

"Christy threw him a curve,—the big, round-house curve that had fooled many a batter in the Virginia League. But the New York manager cracked it on the nose. And as the ball went streaking out over center-field, he said:

" 'That won't do. I could see it coming.'

"He meant that the ball broke,—that is, curved—so early in its flight that he could follow the break with his eye and set himself to hit.

" 'Try this one' said Christy.

"He threw an out-drop which, breaking less widely, broke just before it reached the plate. The manager missed it.

" 'That's better,' he said; 'What else you got?'

"Christy wound up with the same swift, careless motion, but this time the ball did not come like a streak of light. It came so slowly that it seemed to float. The manager checked his swing in time, but just as he chopped at the ball, it faded down and away from him. Reaching for it, he lost his balance and missed it by a foot.

" 'What's that?' he said sharply.

" 'That's the fade-away,' said Christy.

" 'Can you control it?'

" 'Some', said Christy.

"He showed the manager how it was thrown, his wrist turning in instead of out, his palm down instead of up as the ball left his fingers. The motion was the opposite of the natural one, reversing the curve, and because it was against rather than with the natural turn of the wrist, it gave a slow ball with the same wind-up and the same effort as a fast ball. By a twist of the wrist he gained the tremendous pitching asset of a change of pace without the change of motion that would warn the batter. It was, however, extremely difficult to control.

" 'You learn to control that,' the New York Manager said, 'It might be the best thing you got.' "

Perhaps no one who ever pitched won greater control over the ball than Mathewson did. This control, combined with the fact that he always kept in mind the batting qualities, both good and bad, of approximately eighty different players, made it possible for him to deliver the ball at the weakest position for each batter. Even John McGraw, with his knowledge of a batter's weaknesses, during the fourteen years that Mathewson played under his management, left him entirely alone to do his own thinking throughout each game. He said, "Matty knew as much as I did about batters." Cary tells the story of a new recruit to the big league who got three hits off Mathewson that day. His team-mates congratulated him on this astounding feat. But one of them said:

" 'Do you remember what kind of balls Matty gave you for those hits?'

" 'No, said the new recruit, 'Why should I remember?'

" 'Because he will,' said the old timer, 'and he will never give them to you again. You might as well start right in now practising hitting the ball in any and every other place, because that's where he'll put 'em hereafter.' "

In his next twenty times at bat against Mathewson, the new recruit failed to get a single, clean hit.

The first year Mathewson was with the New York Giants he played in only six games and in those he showed no unusual ability; but in the second year, although his team was not strong, he lost seventeen and won twenty games. The following year he won thirty and, in 1904, he lost only twelve and won thirty games. He continued with this great winning ability through 1914. After that his arm began to fail him, but he was a true professional and lost no interest in baseball. He then became manager of the Cincinnati Club.

During the years that he pitched, Mathewson became known to the world as "Matty," "Christy," and "Big Six." He was a man of splendid physique, and his clean living made it possible for him to pitch so long. No one was able to induce him to play ball on Sunday, for he had promised his mother that he never would. Throughout his life, he stood for everything that was uplifting not only in baseball but also in other activities. There were no flaws in his character and no blots on his reputation.

When the United States entered the world war, Mathewson went to France with the "Gas and Flame" division. Here, as in baseball, he threw himself wholeheartedly into his work. He was slightly gassed. Then came influenza. His resistance was reduced. He was never absolutely well after this, although when he returned to America he again took up baseball. For a long time he suffered from "bronchitis" and consulted four different physicians before the real cause of the difficulty was detected. It was tuberculosis. He had believed his trouble of no significance. Indeed, until two days before he began treatment, he was in uniform on the ball field.

As soon as he knew that he was suffering from tuberculosis he went to Saranac Lake, New York; where he became as good a fighter of tuberculosis as he had been a pitcher of baseball. He was terribly ill and his weight fell from more than 200 to less than 150 pounds. The disease was too far advanced to permit of his admission to the Trudeau Sanatorium. He was compelled to secure a house for himself and family where he undertook home treatment. He was so ill that there seemed to be little hope for his recovery and hope waned as his symptoms increased. His death was expected any day and reporters in various parts of the country prepared long obituaries to be used as soon as his death was announced. He lay absolutely quiet in bed and carried out to the letter every order of his physician. The self-control he had practiced and mastered on the baseball diamond became of great value to him in fighting the disease. He lived his motto, "I will surely beat this game." The greater part of his disease was in the left lung, and therefore it was possible to administer artificial pneumothorax. Of the treatment it has been said, "No greater ray of sunshine has ever come to illumine the dark kingdom of disease than that cast in the path of the consumptive through the discovery of artificial pneumothorax." Mathewson continued to follow the advice of the physician and this treatment brought the disease under control.

Mathewson had no illusions about his apparent victory, as is evidenced by his letter to Joe O'Brien, secretary of the New York Giants:

Saranac Lake, February 15, 1921.

"Well Joe, for the first time in twenty-one years, I will not be going South for spring training. Tell John J. (McGraw) that I will surely beat this game; but it will take twelve months longer to do it.

"I sit up in a chair an hour or so nearly every day, and am getting stronger. Now that I am allowed to write letters, I will, of course, write John J."

Concerning this letter and Mathewson's fighting ability, the *Journal of the Outdoor Life*, of April, 1921, comments thus:

"The fact that Matty is resigned to take twelve months longer to beat his game indicates a patience and courage that can come only with a strong character. He has made up his mind to 'stick to it' to 'fight to the finish.' And fighting tuberculosis is a far braver deed than fighting Germans, as Matty did in 1918, or fighting an enemy baseball team. There is nothing spectacular in his fight, no cheering fans in the grandstand, no bands playing, no flying banners and pennants. This is a lonely fight and an uncheered fight. It is a fight full of suffering for the body and for the mind. It is a fight that needs soul strength."

Within a year he was up again. In August, 1922, he was able to go to his home in Factoryville to visit his mother and that same fall he attended the world's series in New York. Within three years from the time his disease was detected he had so completely recovered that he was able to return to work. So, in February, 1923, he became president and part-owner of the Boston Braves, a team which had just purchased the Boston National League Club. During the next two years, although he was active in the work, he was extremely cautious, always consulting his physician before entering into any new activity. He took considerable time for rest and relaxation each summer, and for this he returned to his home in Saranac Lake. All went well and he met with great success. In the spring of 1925 he went to St. Petersburg where the Boston Braves were in training. This trip apparently proved too much for him, and he was soon compelled to return to Saranac Lake. After several months he developed tuberculous pneumonia, and died on October 7, 1925. The news of his death came to the world very unexpectedly, and plunged the whole country into sorrow.

The following is an extract from an editorial

on Mathewson and Johnson, the latter a pitcher for the Washington Senators:

"The same day that saw Walter Johnson pitch the finest game of baseball in all his nineteen American League years, saw Christy Mathewson, ablest pitcher who ever adorned the National League, pass from this life.

"The greatness of these two men cannot be measured in diamond victories alone. The example of the clean-living Mathewson was a wonderful lesson for a whole generation of baseball-loving youngsters. The example of the clean-living Johnson continues the Mathewson tradition.

"No manager ever had to rebuke Christy Mathewson for running around nights, wasting the energy that was needed to win games. No manager has ever had to fine or suspend Walter Johnson for insubordination, or flouting training rules. Both have loved baseball as a painter loves his art. Neither was in the game for the mere money and fame he would garner.

"These are great names, Mathewson and Johnson, names that will live in the hearts of adoring millions."

From far and wide came messages of condolence, thousands of them, to his wife and son.

It seemed that the whole village of Saranac Lake went forth to pay tribute to him. Hundreds gathered around the railroad station as his body was being taken to Mrs. Mathewson's former home in Lewisburg, Pennsylvania. It was in Lewisburg that he had attended Bucknell College and there his son is now a student in the same school. As his body lay in state, multitudes of sorrowing people passed by his bier to pay him their last tribute. Many American baseball notables were in attendance at the funeral. John J. McGraw, Emil Fuchs, David Bancroft, Albert Powell, Edward Reilley and Ernest Sterling were honorary pallbearers. The flags on the Bucknell Campus were lowered to half-staff, and all business in Lewisburg was suspended during the funeral. The death of Mathewson was sincerely mourned throughout the nation, not only because he was the greatest pitcher of modern times and the greatest right-handed pitcher of all times; not only because he won three hundred and seventy-two games as a major league pitcher and for more than sixteen years was premier of the baseball game; but also because he had lived in every respect a clean wholesome life and had justly become the idol of American youth. It has been truthfully said that "boys who try to emulate him as their hero will not go very far wrong."

REFERENCES

Matty's Beating This Game. *Journal of the Outdoor Life*, April, 1921.

"Big Six" New Boss of the Boston Braves. *The Literary Digest*, March 10, 1923.

Mathewson's Biggest Victory. By Lucian Cary. *Good Housekeeping*, August, 1923.

AUBREY BEARDSLEY

AUBREY BEARDSLEY was born at Brighton, England, in 1872 where he received his early education. When only a child he was a lover of music and played the piano exceptionally well. Indeed he has been spoken of as an infant prodigy. While still a child he manifested some aptitude in art, having painted Christmas cards to earn a little spending money. One lady who bought some of these cards wrote Aubrey's mother, thanking her for sending the cards, and adding "I hope your little boy will grow up some day to be a great artist." In 1888 Aubrey illustrated the program and bulletin of the Brighton grammar school annual entertainment. These eleven illustrations were his first published works.

His next drawing was "Hamlet" which appeared in a magazine known as *The Bee* in 1891. At this time Beardsley was working as a clerk in an insurance office. His interest in art was so great that after a full day's work in the office he drew from nine in the evening, his earliest opportunity to do so, until far into the night. Aymer Vallance, having been advised of Beards-

ley's ability, attempted to convince him to devote
his entire life to art. Under Vallance's influence
he studied the human figure, for a short time, in
a studio in Westminister. This, together with a
short period spent in an architect's office constituted his entire education in art. He carried
a portfolio containing his drawings which he
frequently traded to the publishers for books
he desired to own.

At nineteen Beardsley contracted to illustrate
"Morte d'Arthur." At the outset he worked
with great ardor, but after a while his enthusiasm
began to wane so the task became a drudgery.
He was greatly discouraged because of the loss
of detail in his drawings due to the excessive
reductions his publishers insisted upon making.
He even threatened to break his contract because of this situation. His contract called for
a certain number of illustrations each month.
As the end of the month approached none of the
drawings would be ready. Beardsley would
then labor, under great strain, day and night to
complete his distasteful task. Under these conditions he became quite careless, and consequently many of these drawings are inferior to
his usual excellence.

In April, 1893, Mr. Joseph Pennell published
an article on Aubrey Beardsley in *The Studio*,
in which he said:

[233]

"I have lately seen a few drawings which seem to me to be very remarkable. The very limited number which the artist is said to have produced makes their perfection of execution all the more remarkable. I am quite well aware that the mere fact of publicly admitting one's interest in the work of a new man, whose first design may be a delight to artists, is not considered to be good form in criticism. But why should one care about good or bad form,—or criticism, either, for that matter? For the criticism of art today is merely the individual expression of persons who mostly know nothing about their subject.

"But whether Mr. Beardsley's work is appreciated or despised,—and my only fear is that he will suffer from over-appreciation and enthusiasm,—the drawings show decisively the presence among us of an artist, of an artist whose work is quite as remarkable in its execution as in its invention; a very rare combination. It is most interesting to note, too, that though Mr. Beardsley has drawn his motives from every age, and founded his style,—though it is impossible to say what his style may be—on all schools, he has not been carried back into the fifteenth century or succumbed to the limitations of Japan; he has recognized that he is

AUBREY BEARDSLEY

living in the last decade of the nineteenth century, and he has availed himself of mechanical reproduction for the publication of his drawings, which the Japs would have accepted with delight had they but known of it."

Next, Beardsley illustrated "Bon Mots" in a very excellent manner. Then, in 1894, he illustrated "Salome." He did an unheard of thing by using illustrations to ridicule the author. In fact, four of the ten pictures in "Salome" contained caricatures of the writer. This idea proved to be very successful.

Beardsley's next work was in connection with *The Yellow Book*. When this was started he was asked to become its art editor. Although only four numbers of *The Yellow Book* actually contain Beardsley's work, his name became well known through this connection. Next he illustrated the "Rape of the Lock;" and then he began to illustrate "Volpone."

In early life Beardsley's health had been very delicate. He had tuberculosis, and suffered from frequent attacks of hemorrhage. No doubt the disease was made worse by his hard work and irregular hours. In 1896, he had become so ill that he sent a message to Vallance asking him to aid him in the completion of the "Book of Fifty Drawings." Mr. Vallance laid aside his own work to help Beardsley and the manuscript was completed in September of that year.

Despite the presence of advanced tuberculosis, Beardsley continued his work. Indeed he drew the illustrations for "Volpone" until four or five weeks before his death. Vallance says: "Whenever he could, and as long as he could, he worked. The latest drawings, for the illustration of "Mademoiselle de Maupin" and for "Volpone," some of the latter produced only four or five weeks before his death, show no falling off in vigour and inventiveness, but rather a fresh development in technique. It is pitiful to think of him lying prostrate, his active brain teeming with ideas which his poor, wasted hand was unable to express; to think of him asking for pencil and paper, and, after a few unavailing efforts to commit his ideas to definite shape, having to let the pencil drop from his enfeebled fingers."

He spent the winter of 1896 at Bournemouth, where he lived in a house called "Muriel," of which he wrote to a friend: "I feel as shy of my address as a boy at school is of his Christian name when it is Ebenezer or Aubrey." An improvement in his health enabled him to go abroad during the summer. But in the autumn he was sure that hope had been only temporary;

at Mentone he became too ill to work, and he
died in the spring of 1898.

Apparently Beardsley had taken no interest
in religion, until 1897, when he made his first
confession in the Roman Catholic Church.
After his conversion, he said: "I feel now like
someone who has been standing waiting on the
doorstep of a house upon a cold day and who
cannot make up his mind to knock for a long
while. At last the door is thrown open, and
all the warmth of kind hospitality makes glad
the frozen traveler."

It has been said that only a real passion for
art could have enabled Aubrey Beardsley to
compress so much achievement into so short a
space of time. At the begnning of the nineties he was unknown; the decade was little more
than half completed when he died; yet in the
interval he had become the most talked-of
artist in England, and had made for himself a
place in English art which is still notable.

Although Beardsley when a mere boy, was
willing to trade his drawings for books, they
have become very valuable since his death.
In March, 1919, forty-three of his earlier and
slighter works were offered for sale at the Anderson Galleries in New York City. These drawings sold for approximately $7,000.

Symons says: "He had the fatal speed of those who are to die young; that disquieting completeness and extent of knowledge, that absorption of a lifetime in an hour, which we find in those who hasten to have done their work before noon, knowing that they will not see the evening. He had played the piano in drawing rooms as an infant prodigy before, I suppose, he had ever drawn a line; famous at twenty as a draughtsman, he found time, in those incredibly busy years which remained to him, to deliberately train himself into a writer of prose which was, in its way, as original as his draughtsmanship, and into a writer of verse which had at least ingenious and original moments. He seemed to have read everything, and had his preferences as adroitly in order, as wittily in evidence, as almost any man of letters; indeed, he seemed to know more, and was a sounder critic, of books than of pictures; with perhaps a deeper feeling for music than for either. His conversation had a peculiar kind of brilliance, different in order, but scarcely inferior in quality to that of any other contemporary master of that art; a salt, whimsical dogmatism, equally full of convinced egoism and of imperturbable keensightedness."

Raymond says: "Aubrey Beardsley was very typical of the nineties in his unenjoying luxuriousness, his invalid naughtiness, his trammeled originality and pert pessimism. He was, in pictorial art, much that Wilde was in literature, except that he possessed a certain conscience of hand, so to speak, a pride and care for technical quality, which few considerable draughtsmen lack; while Wilde, though an artist also, lacked such fastidiousness and was just as pleased with a cheap victory as with a dear one. Both he and Wilde were in revolt against convention, but each would have died rather than do anything unnaturally. Both were at war with Victorian decorum, but both respected slavishly the little law of a little clique. Both suggested the futility of all things, the one in the most precious prose, the other in the most austerely thought-out design."

In 1919, Pennell wrote: "I wrote *The Studio* article on the faith of the drawings and prints that I was shown, because I knew they were the work of a man, a boy, who had done something to carry on tradition—but I did not know if he would do anything more. And I did know that often such an article is a refuge, a safe harbor for one who can only repeat what he has done and never tries after to go on. But Beardsley was not of that sort—he went on.

"He and Henry Harland started *The Yellow*

Book. I did not believe it would succeed, but it did, and in it Beardsley came into his own. Then, or maybe it was before, he illustrated "Salome;" and then came "The Rape of the Lock," which proved him, as Whistler said, and the world acknowledged, 'a great artist' and won him fame. Then came the "Volpone," and before it was finished came death; but he has built himself an enduring monument. And two boys whom the gods loved, died young—John Keats and Aubrey Beardsley. They died, and from the same cause, but their names and their works live—they are amongst the glorified in English art and letters. Beardsley built better than I knew, but he knew better than I, and it is good to know now that one had a part in those wonderful days in that wonderful world, which is gone, but never will be forgotton."

Although Brehmer and Dettweiler, in Germany, and Trudeau, in America, had demonstrated that tuberculosis can be treated successfully, this knowledge had not been properly disseminated among the public. It was not generally known that tuberculosis is curable. Even today the medical profession is deserving of no more just criticism than that of failing to inform the public of the great advances in medicine. Physicians are so busy diagnosing conditions, treating patients, and advancing technical medical knowledge, that they overlook the fact that before their profession can do the maximum of good to humanity the public also must be well-informed. Had Beardsley and his friends known of the curability of tuberculosis, his life might have been greatly extended. Of this we cannot be absolutely sure, since much depends upon the nervous temperament, etc., of the patient. Even today we see "those who die young" sometimes because they will not submit to the necessary discipline.

Beardsley, having only a few years to work, was greatly handicapped by his tuberculosis, yet the following is truthfully said of him: "No artist of our time, none certainly whose work has been in black and white, has reached a more universal, or a more uncontested fame; none has formed for himself, out of such alien elements, a more personal originality of manner, none has had so wide an influence on contemporary art."

REFERENCES

Aubrey Beardsley. By Arthur Symons.

The Invention of Aubrey Beardsley. By Aymer Vallance. *Magazine of Art*, April, 1919.

An Exhibition of Original Drawings. By Aubrey Beardsley, with a foreword by Joseph Pennell.

Aubrey Beardsley. By E. T. Raymond. *Living Age*, December, 1920.

McDUGALD McLEAN

McDUGALD McLEAN was born on January 20, 1886, at Georgetown, Texas. He was the only child of John and Olivia McDugald McLean. After attending the Webb preparatory school at Bell Buckle, Tennessee, he entered Vanderbilt University. He spent the last three years of his college course at Southwestern University. His popularity with the faculty and student body both in preparatory school and college was attested by the numerous honorary offices which he held.

Under the provisions of the will of Cecil Rhodes the educational facilities of Oxford are available to students in this country who fulfill certain requirements. McDugald McLean's selection by the scholarship committee was unanimous.

In 1910, as the Rhodes scholar from Texas, he entered Christ Church, Oxford, to study pathology and medicine. Here he came in intimate contact with Sir William Osler, "the most widely known and best beloved physician in the world." McLean's experiences with and descriptions of Dr. Osler reveal the reason for the latter's unusual reputation and high regard.

"On this line Dr. Osler (Sir William), represented the nth degree of perfection. Though occupying the exalted position of Regius Professor of Medicine, yet he was the most thoughtful of his students' welfare, kind, helpful, and a real friend. In fact, I believe, he is the only man I ever came in contact with in whom I could find no fault. Wherever he worked his gifted and unique personality was a center of inspiration.

"I was a member of Christ Church College at Oxford, with which Dr. Osler was affiliated. A few days after my first term began he came around to my rooms, said he was Dr. Osler and had just dropped in to see if I was getting started all right, and that if I had no engagements for next Sunday afternoon to drop in at his home for tea.

"Think of the Regius Professor of Medicine at Oxford, and a man as busy as Dr. Osler was, finding time to call on an average "fresher" and welcome him in such a kindly, human way. And those Sunday afternoon teas at his home, with what pleasure I recall them! Often Dr. Osler would come out to the door himself, greet you with a slap on the back, put his arm around your shoulders and lead you into the reception room and introduce you to students, professors, and distinguished men and women from the ends of the earth.

"Dr. Osler offered a course of lectures on the history of medicine. There were only nine of us, I believe, signed up for the course. He gave only two or three lectures during the year, but what a feast they were! We would receive a notice giving the subject of the lecture and the time appointed, and each notice would be accompanied by an invitation to dinner. The lecture would be preceded by a nine-course dinner, the dishes cleared away, cigars and cigarettes passed around, and while we all remained seated around the table Dr. Osler would proceed to give the lecture in an informal manner and conversational tone. Rare old books and pictures would be passed around during the lecture to add interest to the subject under discussion. Who but Dr. Osler would treat his students and the history of medicine in such a unique, interesting, and 'inviting' way?"

One summer vacation McLean spent studying at the University of Freiburg, Germany, attending twenty-two lectures a week. He writes, "I find Freiburg a very pretty place with quite pleasant surroundings. Many good opportunities for day excursions into the Schwarzwald and other such interesting places. There has been a University here since about 1476, I believe, according to Baedeker, and the Medical Department here is third largest in Germany in professors and students—Berlin first, Munich second. They have some very distinguished men here. One among the foremost is Professor Aschoff whose lectures in Pathology I am attending. He is rather small and insignificant looking, but a very hard worker and an excellent lecturer and demonstrator."

One Christmas vacation was spent in Gottingen, Germany, especially for the study of German, but while there McLean attended some clinics. He writes from Gottingen, "I called on Mrs. Landau, a cousin of Hahn's yesterday. She is the daughter of Dr. Ehrlich, the greatest living German doctor, and possibly the greatest living research student in medicine. His theory of Immunity is the one most generally accepted now, and it is the one in accordance with which I am doing my work. Her husband is Professor of Mathematics in the University here, and they have a beautiful large home. She has been in America and knows Dr. Osler quite well."

During his three years at Oxford, Dr. McLean was entertained many times at the home of Sir James Murray. On November 2, 1911, he writes,

"Went to a very interesting Hallowe'en party last Tuesday at Sir James Murray's. He, by the way, is bringing out the *New English Dictionary*, has spent practically his whole life on it, is nearly seventy now I suppose, and is through S, I believe. There are some eight or ten volumes out now; it is published as each volume is completed, and each volume is about the size of a Webster's Unabridged. He is about the wisest mortal I have ever seen—a perfect halo of wisdom shines about him, yet he is very simple in manner and a true unaffected Scotchman. . . . Well, they had looked up all the Hallowe'en games from the flood till now, and we played them—we had a genuine, undignified, childlike good time. . . . The Murrays are about the most informal people I have met over here, a great pleasure and relief occasionally. There are two daughters at home now, who are extraordinarily bright."

The following notice appeared in the *New York Times* August 8, 1915: "The death of Sir James Murray will not prevent the completion of the *New English Dictionary*, the great work upon which he has been engaged as editor for the last twenty-seven years. Happily the labors of the lexicographer, although more arduous today, are better organized than in the days of

Johnson. The death of the latter before his task was finished, would have robbed posterity of the completed results of his researches in philology. The work of Sir James Murray, however, will continue until the final page of his dictionary is reached. The two editors who preceded him, Herbert Coleridge and Dr. Furnivall, accomplished comparatively little, and it looked as if under their new management the dictionary would be abandoned before the publication of its first volume. Sir James Murray's genius for organization insured the success of the enterprise. He had more than 1,500 assistants, whose duty it was to read books, and thirty assistant editors who sorted out the rough material. Every English book published before 1500 A.D. was read, and every book of importance since then. The result was that the work grew more rapidly than the most sanguine had expected. Nine volumes have been published; the tenth and final volume, containing the letters T to Z, remaining incomplete. Its publication will probably not be long delayed."

In another letter Dr. McLean writes, "I have been greatly honored with visitors this past week. The Landaus came over one day and had lunch with us. They brought a friend with them, a Miss Holman-Hunt, and after lunch we went around to see the art gallery and quite suddenly and unexpectedly I discovered that we were in a room where most of the pictures were labeled Holman-Hunt. Thereupon I heard Miss Holman-Hunt remark that 'Father had spent a certain number of months on this picture and that she had not seen it for years.' Shortly thereafter I inquired stealthily of Miss Dorothea Landau if this was the Holman-Hunt who had painted the famous 'Light of the World,' which is now at Keble College, one of the treasures of Oxford, and of course I was greatly impressed when she replied, yes."

Dr. McLean received his Bachelor of Science degree from Oxford. The subject of his thesis was "A Study of Some Factors in Haemolysis."

One of the interesting experiences of Dr. McLean's life was attending the clan gathering of the McLeans of the Isle of Mull. He had had a special invitation from Sir Fitzroy McLean whose lifelong ambition had been to buy Duart Castle that had once belonged to the clan, and replant the standard of the clan on the castle. Upon the realization of this ambition he summoned the McLeans from all over the world to celebrate with him.

Dr. McLean writes from Oban, "We had a great time at the clan gathering yesterday.

About hour hundred McLeans from United States, Canada, Germany, Holland, New Zealand, Australia, England, Ireland and Scotland were here. They came in yachts, motors, trainloads and by foot.

"The Chief summoned me after lunch and I had a most pleasant talk with him and his family. I met fifty awfully nice cousins and three real beauties, etc.—I don't think I have any immediate connections over here now; at least I couldn't trace them very straight as my great-great-grandfather left here about 1750.

"It was a glorious day, perfect weather, the first pretty day for weeks, Good spirits and fellowship abounded, the pipers made the hills echo with Highland tunes, and scores of men were in Highland costume—a picture I shall never forget as long as my cerebrum has one active cell!"

On his return to America he entered upon further study of medicine at Johns Hopkins, and there received the degree of Doctor of Medicine His teachers were a great inspiration to him, especially Dr. Lewellys F. Barker, who was his ideal, and he greatly admired Mrs. Barker too and enjoyed many delightful social occasions in their home. He took advantage of his vacations, as he had abroad, to work with his professors, and also assisting Dr. Barker one summer in the preparation of his book, "The Clinical Diagnosis of Internal Diseases." He also worked with Dr. Styles in Wilmington another summer. He served for one year as interne at the Bay View Hospital at Baltimore before beginning his work as general practitioner. In 1916 he married Miss Emma Webb, daughter of Ex-Senator Webb of Bell Buckle, and went to Dallas, Texas, where he began practicing with the firm of "Baird, Doolittle, Folsom, and McBridge," but almost immediately was taken ill and the trouble was diagnosed tuberculosis. He then went West working for a few months as an assistant in the New Mexico Cottage Sanatorium at Silver City. He was deeply interested in his profession, and was offered many places but was unable to accept them. Toward the end of 1921 his condition became very serious, and in February, 1922, he was confined to his bed and only rarely sat upright.

J. A. Ransom recently wrote of Dr. McLean as follows:

"McLean had a red head and an indomitable spirit. He played a smashing game of tennis (on several occasions he played for the Varsity) and a fine game of golf; his strength seemed greater than that of most men in those days, despite his slight build. He had a huge sense of humor that made a 'rag' the joy of life to him; an unbounded zest for all sorts of games, and for every day of life. He had old fashioned convictions that he was always prepared to defend. He was an idealist, and generous to a fault. These are some scattering qualities that came first as I remember him.

"In his letters he always treated his illness as a joke, and threatened to get up from his sick bed and give me another thrashing at tennis or golf. When I was about to sail for France in 1917, he wrote cursing his luck that he could not go at that time, but promised to get in a few blows at the Kaiser before it was over.

"Mac was the ideal for many Rhodes Scholars, among whom I gladly number myself. He seemed to have just the perfect equipoise of all the qualities that may become a man. He and I were two of a houseful of Scholars that digged together on Walton road during our last year at Oxford, and was the nucleus of many dialectic episodes lasting any time from six-fifteen, or twenty-four hours together. On these occasions he was always the party of the common sense view point; there were some of us who knew very well that we were getting lost in the clouds of speculative philosophy, and that he with his saving humor and his touch with the practical, was the best man in the crowd. Many of us, when it was all over, considered that he was the great man of our year.

"He would have been the superlative doctor of medicine. In spite of his keen faculty for research and specialization, which I believe was very well recognized by his teachers, it was not his intention to shut himself up in a laboratory or a specialty of medicine; he was going to be a general practitioner. In this field his sanity, his humanity, and his science would have made him one of the very few. His wonderful little book, 'Tuberculosis: A Primer and Philosophy for Patient and Public' shows what a rare and inspiring combination of scientific knowledge and human wisdom he would have brought to his profession."

Following is Mrs. McLean's account of the difficulties that Dr. McLean surmounted in the completion of his book. "For several years he had been writing it and from time to time would take it out and add to it and revise it. He was greatly interested in it but never worked on it very long at a time. Suddenly, sometime in May, 1922, he began working on his book with a purpose and resolve he had never seemed to have before. We didn't think he could live to finish it. Since February he had been confined to his bed with frequent attacks of shortness of breath each one of which we thought might be the end. Most of the time after this he kept his typewriter on a little stand we made him across his lap, rewriting many parts of his manuscript. Several times he said to me that he had received inspiration from somewhere, he didn't know where.

"Every detail of bringing out his book was of deep interest to him. He planned everything and wrote many letters. As soon as a letter was written, one of us, my sister or his sister, who were with us, or I, would drop everything and go immediately to the post office and mail it. We had to run on many errands for various phases of the book and in our race with the Angel of Death we allowed nothing to delay us. The mails were of the deepest interest to him and any letter concerning his book was immediately answered by him and mailed by one of us.

"At last the proof was ready and submitted to him for correction. He sent it off in post haste to Dr. Lewellys F. Barker, who was then enjoying a vacation in Canada, feeling that if it had Dr. Barker's approval the success of the book would be assured. Then he grew anxious—fears and doubts came into his mind, fear of embarrassing Dr. Barker and doubts of the real value of his book.

"One day while the doctor was there because of Dr. McLean's serious condition, the postman arrived at the door. I took the mail to his room and told him he had a letter. 'Open it and see who it is from' he said. I told him it was from Dr. Barker and began reading it aloud. 'Don't read it aloud,' he directed. 'But, Dugald,' I said, 'It is too good to keep—I must read it to you now.' I couldn't let him go without hearing the good news. Then I read him a beautiful letter from Dr. Barker, his superman, freely according it recognition and beautiful words of praise. His face was radiant and his breathing grew stronger. He lived about two months after this.

"Soon afterward the book was finished—he did a little advertising and he began getting numbers of orders that pleased him tremendously. As soon as an order came we filled it, and many letters of appreciation reached him before the end, letters that made him realize his book was a success."

Dr. McLean's book, "Tuberculosis: A Primer and a Philosophy," was published in 1922. In it are laid down not only the principles necessary for recovery, but also the principles necessary for the prevention of the disease. All through the book one is conscious of his far reaching vision into the field of preventive medicine. In discussing prevention and education in the preface he says: "When every one is thoroughly awake to the situation that tuberculosis can be more *easily* and *successfully* and *cheaply prevented* than *cured*, a big advance toward this end has been made." In this book he deals with such subjects as selfishness, ignorance, and undue fear on the part of the patient, relatives, and friends. In his chapter on "Good and Bad Advice" he deals a lasting blow to those persons offering advice regarding a disease about which they know nothing. He says, "All shades and qualities of advice can be had for the asking—and often without the asking. Ignorance of the issues at stake does not restrain these voluble advisers from proffering their well-meant but misdirecting and meddlesome advice with great assurance and insistence. Ne'er-do-wells and failures in all walks of life are notorious advisers. One danger from such advice is the tendency to accept it when it coincides with our whims and pleasure in preference to the best advice, which may not be so convenient and pleasant to take."

In another chapter he points out that morale is just as important a factor for the patient as it is for the soldier. In this chapter he discusses serenity, religion, philosophy, physiological effect of emotions, cause of depressive emotions, self-control, evil effects of worry, etc.

In speaking of the chapter on "Health vs. Patent Medicine, Charlatans and Christian Science," Mr. James Hay, Jr. says, "But it is on the subject of patent medicine, charlatans and fake 'cures' of the disease that the doctor throws off all restraint and with obvious pleasure un-limbers the heavy guns of his sarcasm, invective, and denunciation. Anybody who delights in the cutting phrase and the hammer-like exposi-tion of the fact is respectfully referred to the chapter in which he treats of those persons and things."

In a special chapter the subject of climate and altitude is treated in a very fair manner. Having been a physician treated in several differ-ent places, Dr. McLean was in a position to write authoritatively on this subject. His advice is as follows: "To sum up the best advice on climate and altitude, I would repeat that they are not essentials in the treatment of tuberculosis. It is agreed that the proper management and supervision of a patient is vastly more important than climate. However, if one can avail himself of its favorable influence without too great a sacrifice of finances and too great a disturbance of his mental equilibrium consequent upon the separation from his family, friends, etc., and can be assured that he will be as carefully looked after in the new environment as in the old, it is certainly advisable for him to make the change."

Of this book the *British Journal of Tuberculosis* says, "The book is addressed primarily to American readers, but we would commend it to the consideration not only of patients in this country, but to medics and others who are working to carry out anti-tuberculosis work by educational measures."

Realizing to the utmost because of his excellent training and native intelligence what the future held for him, Dr. McLean had forged on, unflinching, to the end of his task. Like Laennec he understood perfectly what the inevitable outcome of the battle must be, and like Laennec, he died fighting. By his death on September 8, 1922, at Asheville, North Carolina, the tuberculosis campaign suffered irreparable loss. To measure length of life in this world from the standpoint of contribution and service to humanity, is better than to measure by length of years. By this standard McDugald McLean lived to be exceedingly old.

REFERENCES

The Journal of the Outdoor Life, December, 1922.
Texas Christian Advocate, October 12, 1922.
Personal communications from Mrs. McLean.

HAROLD BELL WRIGHT

HAROLD BELL WRIGHT, the second of the four sons of William Wright and Alma Watson Wright, was born on May 4, 1872, in Rome, New York. He was left an orphan at the age of ten, with the necessity of shifting for himself. He spent the next five years in doing odd jobs, and especially in training himself for the position of house-painter and decorator. He had no intention of remaining at work with his hands, and at the age of twenty he entered the preparatory department of Hiram College, in Ohio. In order to secure the necessary funds while in school he did odd jobs of house-painting and decorating about the town. But, after two years, he suffered a severe attack of pneumonia which cut short the schooling, and sent him to the Ozark Mountains, in southwestern Missouri, in search of health. While gradually regaining his strength, he put in his time painting and sketching, for he had decided to become an artist.

One night he attended "meetin" in a little schoolhouse. The minister failed to appear, and the congregation having come from long distances was loathe to depart without a service of some kind. One of the deacons approached Mr. Wright and said, "You look like an educated man. Will you preach to us?" Mr. Wright protested that preaching was hardly in his line, but he agreed to talk. The congregation liked his little sermon so well that they kept him as preacher all winter.

In the meantime, Mr. Wright kept up his work of painting; but he began to feel more and more drawn to the ministry. When he was offered a regular pastorate at Pierce City, Missouri, at a salary of four hundred dollars a year, he accepted. A little later he received a call from a church in Pittsburgh, Kansas, and at the same time an exceedingly tempting offer of work as a commercial artist. He felt that he could do more good in the ministry, so he accepted the call. While at Pittsburgh, he wrote his first story, "That Printer of Udell's." It was written without thought or intention of offering it for publication, but to be read, in installments, on certain evenings to his congregation. Some of his friends, however, persuaded him to offer it for publication, so that its message might reach beyond his congregation to the rest of the world.

From Pittsburgh he was called to Kansas City where he remained for a year. After a severe

attack of grip Mr. Wright's physician told him
that while he did not have active tuberculosis,
"the ground is well prepared and ready for the
seed." With his family he moved to southern
California and settled on a ranch in the Imperial
Valley.

Mr. Wright had finished "The Shepherd of
the Hills" before coming to California. Now in
his open air study, in the Imperial Valley he
wrote "The Calling of Dan Matthews" and then
"The Winning of Barbara Worth," the latter
probably his best known novel, which sold up
to more than two million copies. "Their Yes-
terdays" (1912) followed, and then "The Eyes
of the World" (1914), his first novel to be produced as a moving picture.

Then came the accident which nearly ended
Mr. Wright's life. His own story of "Why
I Did Not Die" is as thrilling and remarkable a
tale as anyone of his own novels.

With a friend he was riding home from El Cen-
tro one day, enjoying the beautiful country,
when suddenly a car roared up behind them,
struck the horse of Mr. Wright's friend, throwing
the horse into the air, and the rider fell with
such force on the hard road that he was rendered
unconscious, although not seriously injured.
The machine then jerked to the right, crashing

into Mr. Wright's horse, throwing the frightened animal into a barbed wire fence. The
corner of the windshield struck Mr. Wright's
left side. The horse miraculously did not go
down, but horse and rider were carried for a
hundred feet along the torturing barbed wire
before the automobile cleared them and came
to a stop.

At first, Mr. Wright did not seem to be in
much pain. He was able to dismount and walk
back to his companion, and not until he reached
up to lift the saddle from the horse did he realize
how badly he was hurt. Fortunately the accident was seen by a neighbor who was behind
them in a car, for the driver of the car which
struck them continued on his journey unconcerned. Besides the injury to the left side of
his chest, caused by the windshield, Mr. Wright
was bruised from waist to foot, and was injured
in the abdomen by the horn of the saddle when
his horse reared.

After a few weeks, Mr. Wright moved to Los
Angeles, where they had planned to make their
home. For months he was constantly under
the physician's care because of a steadily increasing pain in his left side. The injury to the abdomen did not give him so much trouble. He
could scarcely walk a hundred yards without

bringing on a terrible attack of coughing. He tried to work, as he had a novel which had been promised for the coming spring, but the writing went very slowly.

Finally, after a thorough examination, Mr. Wright was told that he had active tuberculosis. His first reaction to this information, he said, was one of *relief*. At last the fight was to be in the open; he knew exactly who and what the enemy was. He decided to go to Tucson, Arizona, and wasted no time in ordering a complete camping outfit to be shipped to Tucson at once. He also hired a negro man and his wife, who professed to be experts at camp life, to do the cooking and to take care of the camp.

The trip to Tucson was a hard one and the effort of getting the camp located, combined with a hard cold, sent Mr. Wright to the hospital for a lonely Christmas. When he was well enough to go to the camp, he found that the two "expert" campers had not succeeded in even getting the tents up. This was accomplished, with Mr. Wright directing operations although he was too weak to actually assist.

No sooner were the tents set up than the dry, mild climate of Arizona belied the fact by rain. There followed day after day of cold and wind and rain, and Mr. Wright sat, huddled in

[263]

his tent, and wondered if he could hold on. The returns from the projected book would provide for his family and for the education of his three sons, for the advance orders were already large enough to insure its success. The book was to be finished the first of May. He was unable to write until the first of February and then for short periods only. Mr. Wright realized the necessity of conserving all his strength, and of never crossing the line of exhaustion, so he rested frequently.

Finally the rain was over and the sunshine came. With the passing of the storms went the two colored "experts" and in their place came a Japanese boy, who cooked things which Mr. Wright could eat, instead of the rich greasy foods the darkies delighted in. The sun continued to shine and Mr. Wright began to gain in strength, the cough ceased, and although he was careful not to overdo, his working capacity gradually increased.

In order that the healing sunlight might reach him in its purest state he bought a complete outfit of white clothing. He fixed a writing table, with a hood to shield his eyes from the glare on the white paper, and worked while he took sun treatments.

To fight off his periods of depression, he made

friends with the wild creatures that were about him, knowing how unwise it is to dwell on oneself and one's troubles. "Most sick people," says Mr. Wright, "are continually digging themselves up to see if they are growing. Give yourself a chance. Let yourself mentally alone. Go away with your thoughts, somewhere, and leave yourself behind. There is no rest for the one who thinks about his troubles all the time. There is no hope for the one who eats his heart out in self-pity."

"If you have nothing to think about, *find* yourself something,—*anything*,—rattlesnakes, Gila monsters, birds, flowers, the stars. Oh! the world is full of interesting things. If it is not, why should you wish to stay here? If you can't find anything to think about except yourself, you ought to die, on general principles,— and you probably will."

Mr. Wright's publisher visited him to see the progress of his book. The manuscript of "When a Man's a Man" was ready for the printers on the last day of April. Five months before, he had thought it would be his last book. Since then he has planned thirteen, among them "The Re-Creation of Brian Kent," "Helen of the Old House," and "The Mine with the Iron Door," the last a romance of the Catalina Mountains in Arizona, where Mr. Wright recovered his health.

Mr. Wright has been asked, "Am I really well, as well as I used to be?" And his reply: "I can ride a horse thirty or forty miles at a stretch and, if the occasion demands, I can ride him hard. I drive a car anywhere a car can go. I swim. I walk all day, hunting or prospecting. I climb hills. I work on ten- or twelve-hour stretches if I wish. *But*—I know there is a limit, over which I must not go. The horse I ride must be gentle. No more bronchos for me! No more taking a hand in the round-ups! No more roping wild horses! When my car is stuck in the mud or sand I take time to use my head and don't try to pull it out by main strength. I swim but little; mostly I sit on the edge of the pool and enjoy seeing the others do their stuff. I tramp leisurely when hunting. I climb slowly, with frequent rests, and visit the higher peaks only on horseback or via my field glasses. I work; but realizing that health is my capital, I try to use judgment in investing it."

And Mr. Wright sums up his experience thus: "The first thing you must do is to *face the facts*. Get your trouble out into the open and look at it squarely. Do not deceive yourself. Do not permit others to deceive you. Show your doctor that he can trust you with the truth.

"There is a lot of shallow talk about pessimism and optimism. Again I say: 'Face the facts.' It is not pessimism to recognize the fact that you cannot live at the bottom of the sea like an oyster! To assert that you can is not optimism—it is foolishness.

"Don't exaggerate your trouble, and don't belittle it; for these are the two sides of the same ditch. An exact, clear-eyed examination of the facts, with an impersonal, cool-headed estimate of the situation,—this is where you must begin. Having done this you can then with intelligence set yourself to get well."

REFERENCES

Harold Bell Wright: A Biography. Elsbery W. Reynolds.

Harold Bell Wright: The Man Behind the Novels. By Hildegarde Hawthorne.

The Personality of Harold Bell Wright. By Bailey Millard.

"Why I did not die." By Harold Bell Wright, American Magazine, June, 1924.

ROGER W. BABSON

ROGER *W*. BABSON was born July 6, 1875, in Gloucester, Massachusetts. As a boy he was industrious to the extent of working while other boys played. Inspired by the talks of his father, who was a merchant, Babson engaged in the business of selling fresh vegetables from house to house.

Mr. Babson studied civil engineering at the Massachusetts Institute of Technology, receiving the degree of Bachelor of Science in 1898. His first position was to examine the properties of traction companies whose securities the banker, his employer, handled. Two years after graduation, he married Miss Grace Margaret Knight of St. Paul.

In the autumn of 1902, while he was engaged in investigations, he contracted a severe "cold." This "cold" developed into an illness, which he fought well into the winter. Babson is not the sort of man whose questions could be evaded indefinitely, and his repeated demands of, "What is the matter with me?" finally got the truth. His physician and his wife told him, as gently as possible, that he had advanced tuberculosis which had already destroyed one lung and had attacked the other. To most people this diagnosis brings great discouragement, but Mr. Babson, far from being stunned, was considerably relieved to know the true cause of his illness. Having found the trouble he went forth with great determination to cure it. His sole business in life just then was to recover his health. He was an excellent patient; he followed his physician's orders to the letter; complete rest, plenty of nourishment, good ventilation and medical supervision were employed. Babson and his wife went West. He was determined to live, and because he backed up his determination with a scientific, methodical pursuit of health, he did live.

Merely living, however, was not sufficient. There was nothing the matter with his brain, and to Babson an idle body in no wise meant an idle mind. To provide for his wife as well as for himself was still his problem in spite of his illness. His old bank position was no longer open to him because he must live absolutely in the open air. He must do nothing that required physical exertion, yet work in the open seemed to mean physical exertion. He had orders to live in the West, but the East drew him through family and business ties. The problem was too complicated for solution.

Babson did the impossible. He decided that there was quite as much fresh air on the Atlantic as on the Pacific Coast; that if he was willing to endure the discomfort of living out-of-doors in a cold climate, the East would serve as well as the West for a place of residence. In this point his views were in advance of those of the medical profession, since at that time the belief was generally held that climatic change is essential to restoration of health and that one must forever after live in the climate where health had been restored. Consequently, Babson and his wife moved back to Wellesley Hills.

Slowly he gained strength although it was a long and tedious task. Meanwhile the maintenance problem was as troublesome as in the West. His active brain was still interested in the monthly reports of railroads and other companies because of his previous occupation.

Finally this thinking and reading bore definite fruit. Babson realized that many bank clerks did exactly what he had been doing, each for his own particular institution, which meant needless duplication and expense. Why not have that analysis and tabulation made by one man instead of several? Why could not he be *the one* man to do it? He could receive reports, analyze them, tabulate them, send them to a group of banks, and divide the expense among them. He could do this in his open air bedroom quite as satisfactorily as at a desk in a bank.

His letters explaining the scheme brought a satisfactory reply from eight banks. Each agreed to pay twelve dollars and fifty cents a month for the service. Thus was started one of the now famous business services of the country.

Steadily the business grew. The house next door was used for offices. Later these were moved to a business back in Wellesley Hills. Babson's strength increased along with his business and his vision broadened. His original service of "Collecting and Selling" business statistics developed into a "Composite Circular of Bond Offerings." He found there were thousands of unlisted bond issues not quoted in financial reports. One seller or one buyer had no way of knowing what the other sellers were asking or what other buyers were paying. The result was that some buyers paid as much as ten points more than others were paying, in the same city, for the same bonds.

When Mr. Babson announced that he was going to list these thousands of bonds, with the names of the owners who wanted to sell, and of the persons wishing to buy, together with the prices at which sales were made, people laughed at him and said it could not be done. He made this idea into a reality, as he had done before. His next development was the "Babson Stock and Bond Description" which revolutionized the old system of supplying information relative to corporations.

Later, he sold both these services, which still are carried on by their present owners, and devoted his time and energy to the "Babson Reports." He bought control of the Moody Manual Company and established the Babson Statistical Organization, which is today the largest business of its kind in the world. The main offices of this organization, of which he is now president, are located in Wellesley Hills, but branch offices are to be found in twenty-six American cities.

All of this expansion inevitably called for larger quarters and Mr. Babson erected a large four-story brick building in Wellesley Hills. His idea that a large clearing-house of financial information could be located outside of a city was ridiculed. A second and still larger building has now been erected to meet the demands of the constant enlargement.

During the war, he worked for the government in connection with the Department of Labor, in Washington. The ultimate outgrowth of this work was the Babson Institute, for the training of business executives. This is the last phase of the development he has projected.

Most of his spare time is spent working on a tract of land which he purchased outside of Wellesley Hills. Here he does such labor as clearing out underbrush, cultivating his garden and packing apples. His house is carefully planned to answer his requirements. The porch upon which he sleeps, the year around, is built in two parts; one enclosed, the other open. The beds are kept in the enclosed porch throughout the cold winter days; and are rolled out at night, warm and comfortable.

Mr. Babson's positions evidence his worth. He is Vice-President of the Newton Trust Company, The Adirondack Light and Power Company and the Hudson Mohawk Company. He is a director of the New Mexico and Arizona Land Company, The Mississippi River Power Company and The Eastern Massachusetts Street Railway Company. He has been made a Fellow of the Royal Statistical Society (London). He is widely and favorably known as a lecturer on statistics and economics. In addition Mr. Babson is author of "Business Barometers," "Selected Investments," "Bonds and Stocks," "Commercial Papers," "The Future of the Working

Classes," "The Future of World Peace," "The Future of the Churches," "The Future of the Nations," "The Future Method of Investing Money," and "The Future of South America."

It is true that one who has had personal experience with any disease can do, during convalescence and after the restoration of working capacity, a tremendous amount of good in the campaign against it. Indeed such ex-patients are often capable of wielding greater influence than physicians and nurses. Mr. Babson is deeply interested in the promotion of good health, not only in his own family, but also among his employees. He is waging a war against disease by issuing a series of health bulletins containing pertinent suggestions in regard to proper living and prevention of disease. These bulletins are included in the worker's pay envelopes. Tuberculosis, naturally, is often the subject of the bulletin.

Thus Mr. Babson, suffering from advanced tuberculosis, defeated the disease, and while fighting the decisive battle conceived an idea which, well-applied, placed him in the foremost rank of American business men. Moreover, while fighting the disease he gained an experience which he is now using to good advantage in the prevention of sorrow, suffering and untimely death among his fellow men. He has a good working capacity at the present time and his life is an outstanding example of what can be accomplished by the tuberculous patient, not only from the standpoint of the restoration of his own working capacity, but also from the heights of great achievement in the fields of service.

REFERENCES

A Man Who Refused to be "As Good As Dead." *American Magazine*, February, 1920. Who's Who in America, 1924–1925.
The Story of Roger W. Babson's Double Battle. *The Journal of the Outdoor Life*, June, 1920

LAWRASON BROWN

THERE came to Saranac Lake, in 1898, a young man suffering from pulmonary tuberculosis who was destined to play an active part in shaping the policies of the Trudeau Sanatorium and to become one of the world's most notable physicians. This young man was Lawrason Brown. He was born in Baltimore on September 29, 1871. After receiving his preliminary education in the schools of Baltimore, he entered the Johns Hopkins University taking the degree of Bachelor of Arts, in 1895. He was determined to study medicine and entered the Johns Hopkins Medical School. While still a medical student, in the third year of the course, he developed pulmonary tuberculosis. He went to Paul Smith's where he became acquainted with the already famous Trudeau. Here an association developed which has been productive of much good to the world. His health was sufficiently restored that he was able to complete the work for the degree of Doctor of Medicine, graduating in 1900 from the Johns Hopkins Medical School.

Dr. Trudeau saw in Dr. Brown very unusual

possibilities, and, in 1900, made him assistant
resident physician to the sanatorium. He had
held this place only one year when he was promoted to the position of head resident physician.
This put him in charge of the medical work and
gave him a wonderful opportunity to become
familiar with all phases of the treatment of
tuberculosis. In his autobiography, Dr. Trudeau writes of Dr. Brown as follows: "The
essential factors of the sanitarium method of
treating tuberculosis I had labored to demonstrate practically, in the face of much opposition
and many difficulties, with such devoted medical
help and with such limited resources as I could
secure throughout the first fifteen years of the
sanitarium's existence. It took all my energies
for many years, however, merely to keep the
institution afloat long enough to demonstrate
by practical results the great truths for which
it stood. These were all generally accepted
and permanently established when Dr. Brown
became Resident Physician, but the methods
were crude, the discipline imperfect, and the
records incomplete. The simple and efficient
rules of discipline; the thorough instruction of
physicians, nurses and patients; the accurate
medical reports and the exhaustive post-dis-
charge records of all patients since the institu-

tion started; the Medical Building, with its facilities for the careful study of all cases on admission, and another scientific laboratory, all sprang
into life as a result of Dr. Brown's insistent
efforts for efficiency and continued progress.

"As I had been only too glad to turn over the
Laboratory in Saranac Lake to Dr. Baldwin, it
was an immense relief to place the medical department of the sanitarium entirely in Dr.
Brown's hands, since, soon after his arrival,
my health and my capacity for work began
steadily to fail."

In 1912, Dr. Brown opened an office in Saranac Lake for private practice and consultation
work. Then he became consulting physician
to the sanatorium. After this Dr. Trudeau said,
"I still have his friendly counsel and help to
turn to."

Dr. Brown has always taken advantage of
opportunities to do educational work, not only
for the members of his profession, but also for
patients, and others interested in tuberculosis.
While a resident physician at the sanatorium,
in 1903, he founded *The Journal of the Outdoor
Life* and edited it for nine years. Perhaps while
struggling with this journal in its beginning he
did not completely realize the great good he was
accomplishing. Nevertheless, he continued his

untiring efforts through the years and, in 1912, he allowed a committee of the National Tuberculosis Association to take it over and continue its publication. Under the splendid management of Dr. Philip P. Jacobs *The Journal of the Outdoor Life* continues to be one of the most efficient health magazines in existence. Its pages carry some of the best and most authoritative articles ever written on various phases of tuberculosis and closely allied subjects. These articles are written in such simple English that not only the physician, but also the patient may clearly understand them. Each month this journal carries a wonderful message to the thousands who read it. The beginning of all this success, and much more, we owe to Dr. Lawrason Brown.

For some years Dr. Brown has been a member of the editorial staff of *The American Review of Tuberculosis*, a monthly periodical which, under the able editorship of Dr. Allen K. Krause, has become the foremost medical journal, devoted to tuberculosis, in the world.

Perhaps no book ever written for tuberculous patients has had a wider sale or served a longer period of usefulness than Dr. Brown's "Rules for Recovery from Tuberculosis." This book is already in its fourth edition. It contains all the information the patient needs and is especially valuable to ex-sanatorium patients. This book should be in the possession of not only every tuberculous patient, but of every physician and tuberculosis worker.

Dr. Brown has written more than eighty-eight articles for journals, twenty-five of which are for the practitioners of medicine. Perhaps more than to anyone else the tuberculosis workers of this country look to Dr. Brown's work for help and guidance. He has that rare ability of taking a complex subject, analyzing it and expressing it in such terms as to make it readily intelligible to the medical reader in general. No better example of this is to be found than in his work on the diagnosis of pulmonary tuberculosis which appeared a few years ago in *The Journal of the American Medical Association*. The pioneer work which he did recently on intestinal tuberculosis in collaboration with H. L. Sampson marks one of the great advances in our knowledge of that phase of tuberculosis, not only from the standpoint of detection but also of treatment. This work which Dr. Brown regards as his best has recently been elaborated and published in book form under the title of "Intestinal Tuberculosis—Diagnosis and Treatment." Already it has led to the prevention of much suffering and the saving of many lives. His "Theses—Diagnostic, Prognostic, and Therapeutic" are classics. They are known everywhere. Not only are they known, but they are used. Besides the large number of articles which he has written for current journals, Dr. Brown has been called upon to contribute chapters to some of the leading textbooks of medicine, as, for example, Osler's "Modern Medicine," and Tice's "System of Medicine." He is also editor of the section of diseases of the chest exclusive of the heart and great vessels in the "Year Book of Medicine," published in Chicago.

In addition to the large amount of time Dr. Brown gives to the individual instruction of patients and physicians, he is a member of the faculty of the famous Trudeau Post-Graduate School of Tuberculosis and takes an important part in the education of physicians who fill this school to capacity each year. It has been the great privilege of many physicians to take his course of lectures and no one has done so without realizing their large value.

At an early date, Dr. Brown began to gather a great tuberculosis library. In a recent article, under the title of "Personal Recollections," he says, "The Sanatorium gave these workers their board, and paid some of them, while I doled out to the others enough to enable them to exist. This made some inroads in my income, which was usually spent about as fast as it came in for my medical library. The sanatorium had no medical library and took no medical journals. The library at the Saranac Laboratory was well supplied with journals and scientific books, but was lacking in clinical works. About this time the first tuberculosis exhibit was held under the auspices of Dr. Osler and his Baltimore confrères. Dr. Welch drew up a list of the one hundred best books on tuberculosis, and, as I had always been a lover of books and a collector in a small way, my desire was of course to acquire them all. Being early in the field I nearly achieved my ambition and for years afterward added nearly every work of any clinical importance."

After gathering this extensive private collection Dr. Brown recently gave it to the library of the Trudeau Sanatorium. In this gift he evidenced once more his wonderful spirit by making this rare group of books and periodicals available to a large number of present and future workers in tuberculosis.

As the years have passed, demands upon Dr. Brown's time have increased, since his very extensive studies and his thorough training have

prepared him for the highest of positions of
service. He has become President of the Medical Board as well as a trustee of the Sanatorium.
He is also trustee of the New York State Sanatorium at Bay Brook, New York. Many other
notable honors have been bestowed upon him
by the members of his profession. He has been
elected to membership in the American Medical
Association, Association of American Physicians,
The American Clinical and Climatological Association, The American Association for Thoracic
Surgery, The American Public Health Association and numerous other organizations. He has
served as the President of the American Clinical
and Climatological Association.

Dr. Brown was especially instrumental in the
creation of the American Sanatorium Association, organized in 1905. The object of this
association is "to promote the professional and
social relations of the members and to advance
the knowledge of the sanatorium treatment of
pulmonary tuberculosis." The original group,
consisting of nineteen members has grown into
a strong and influential association of more than
two hundred which has rendered a large service
to sanatorium interests. Dr. Brown has held
various offices in this organization, including its

Presidency, and it may be fairly said that his has been the chief guiding hand in its development.

From 1918 to 1919, Dr. Brown served as Vice-President of the National Tuberculosis Association and, in 1922, the greatest honor that can come to any tuberculosis worker in this country was his when he was elected its President.

Like Dr. Trudeau, Dr. Brown has taken great interest in affairs outside the realm of his profession. For example, he was the first president of the Adirondack Good Roads Association. The good macadam roads running through the Adirondacks, which Dr. Trudeau mentions in his autobiography, are in no small part due to his efforts. He was also the first president of the Stevenson Society of America.

When one considers his great contributions in the past; when one recognizes his continuing capacity for work, excelled by no one in his profession today; when one realizes that there is now no greater living producer of the excellent in medical literature; and when one remembers that all of this has been and is being done by one who suffered from clinical tuberculosis more than twenty-five years ago and has been none too well on several occasions since; one grows well convinced that the tuberculous patient may,

nevertheless, ascend to the heights of his chosen
vocation or profession.

REFERENCES

An Autobiography. By Edward Livingston Trudeau.
A History of The National Tuberculosis Association.   S. A. Knopf.
Rules for Recovery from Tuberculosis.   By Lawrason Brown.
The Journal of the Outdoor Life, January, 1925.

WILL IRWIN

WILL IRWIN was born in Oneida, New York, on September 14, 1873, of old American ancestry, derived from the English and Scotch. John Greene, his earliest American maternal ancestor, went with Roger Williams to found Rhode Island in the thirties of the seventeenth century. His paternal ancestors came from Scotland in the colonial period.

Lured by the untold possibilities in the gold strike and the mining prospects, David Irwin went West to Leadville, Colorado, then at the height of the greatest mining boom of the decade. A year later he sent for his wife and sons, Wallace and Will, the latter being then about five or six years old. The journey was made by train as far as Denver and thence by stage-coach through the Rockies up to the very top of the continental divide where Leadville was situated.

Leadville is one of the glowing romances of the early period, for it was the wildest mining camp of this time. It was also the richest mining camp, but the Irwin's fortune did not prosper accordingly. Will as a result, overtaxed his strength in attempting to eke out the family finances. Besides attending school, he arose at four o'clock in the morning in order to distribute the daily newspapers, on horseback, among the mines. He "punched cattle" one summer under the now vanishing conditions of the "open range."

The family moved to Denver when Will was fifteen. Graduating from the West Denver High School, he worked at odd jobs for the next two years. At one time he was the member of a company of "barnstorming" actors, in the fashion of the Jitney Players of today, but the company went into bankruptcy in Kansas.

Entering Leland Stanford in the class of 1898, he worked his way through the university, with the aid of some borrowed money, as the head-waiter in the dormitory. Herbert Hoover was also working his way as a laundry agent, at this time. Irwin developed his literary talents by writing a large amount of verse and by producing, as well as writing, most of the college theatricals. He was the author of a song satirizing the faculty that was very popular with the students in a surreptitious manner. The faculty learned of it in the last term of Irwin's senior year and expelled him. He was given his degree, in absentia, a year later.

Irwin's first position, as a reporter, was on the San Francisco *Wave*. His predecessor was Frank Norris, the novelist, and he later succeeded J. O'Hara Cosgrave, as editor. When the *Wave* was discontinued after a year and a half's time, Irwin became the star reporter on the *San Francisco Chronicle*. During this time he wrote his first novels in collaboration with Gelett Burgess.

In 1904 he accepted the position as star reporter on the New York *Sun*. In 1906 he became managing editor; later editor-in-chief of *McClure's Magazine*, a leading American popular periodical. He left *McClure's* after a year's time to go into free lance writing. Numerous articles by him appeared in *Collier's*, in *Everybody's*, and principally in the *Saturday Evening Post*. Simultaneously with this magazine he was engaged in writing his novels.

His decision to give up reporting entirely was shattered by the outbreak of the World War. On August 6, 1914, less than a week after Germany invaded Belgium, he was on his way to Europe. Exactly twelve days after that, he was a prisoner of war in the hands of the Germans, with three other American correspondents attached to the Belgian army who had gone through the Belgian lines and encountered the

Germans at Louvain. After a fortnight of adventure, which included a forbidden visit to the German front during the battle of Mons, he crossed the Dutch border. The next four and a half years he served as a war correspondent in four countries, returning to America every year in the middle of the winter. He wrote, during the early part of the war, for several American periodicals and the London *Times*, but in the latter part, exclusively for the *Saturday Evening Post*. In 1918 the United States Government called him back to Washington to organize the foreign propaganda. He spent several strenuous months at this work. Upon returning to Europe he was attached to the American Army for the remainder of the war and during the peace conference.

Besides the herculean labours Irwin accomplished as a correspondent, he wrote two novels during the war. The discussions preliminary to the disarmament conference inspired his next book, "The Next War," an attempt to show the gigantic folly of war under the present organization of society. The book had an immense vogue and is his best seller to date. It led him to two seasons on the lecture platform.

Early in 1916, he came back from the war to marry Inez Haynes Gillmore of literary fame.

Mrs. Irwin is the author of the following books: "June Jeopardy," 1908; "Maida's Little Shop," 1910; "Phoebe and Ernest," 1910; "Janey" 1911; "Phoebe, Ernest and Cupid," 1912; "Angel Island," 1914; "The Ollwant Orphans," 1915; "The Californiacs," 1916; "The Lady of Kingdoms," 1917; "The Happy Years," 1919; "The Native Son," 1919; "The Story of the Woman's Party," 1921; "Out of the Air," 1921; "Maida's Little House," 1921; and "Gertrude Haviland's Divorce" 1925. She was a founder, with Maud Wood Park, of the National College Equal Suffrage League; and is a member of the Advisory Council of the National Woman's Party. In 1925, she won the O'Henry prize, given annually for the best American short story.

Mr. Irwin received such honors and decorations as that of the Chevalier of the Legion of Honor, the King Albert medal, first class, The Medaille de la Reconnaissance, and the Commemorative Medal of the Olympic games.

Irwin's life story is that of an exceedingly energetic and healthy human being. Yet at the age of nineteen Dr. Dennison, a tuberculosis specialist of Denver, diagnosed his "severe cold" as tuberculosis. The microscopic examination of the sputum, although this was not long after the initial discovery of the tubercle bacillus by

Koch, as well as the physical examination, substantiated this diagnosis. At this time no sanitary precautions whatsoever were taken. Denver was crowded with tuberculous patients ordered there for the supposed salutary effects of the altitude and dry climate, and permanent residents may have contracted the disease from these migratory consumptives.

At this time Trudeau was struggling with the establishment of his sanatorium in the Adirondacks. The idea of rest treatment in tuberculosis was not widely disseminated and patients were commonly advised to live a hardy outdoor life. Following out this advice, Irwin went to work on a ranch in the early winter, and the following fall was working in the hay fields. He regained most of his weight and the physician pronounced the disease arrested. Since his doctor strongly condemned the New England climate, Irwin abandoned the plan to attend Harvard and entered Stanford. Although he played football for one season at Stanford; went through the World War, receiving a ruptured ear drum from a bursting shell at Caperetto; was gassed at the second battle of Ypres; and had a severe attack of "flu," during the period of the great epidemic; and worked almost incessantly at all other periods of his life, he has never had a recurrence

[291]

of tuberculosis. Ever since his illness, Irwin
has made a special effort to keep himself in good
physical condition and to this fact he attributes
his apparently perfect health for the last
thirty years.

He is the author of "Stanford Stories" (with
C. K. Field), 1900; "The Reign of Queen Isyl"
(with Gelett Burgess), 1903; "The Picaroons"
(with Gelett Burgess), 1902; "The Hamadryads"
(verse), 1904; "The City That Was," 1907;
"Old Chinatown," 1908; "The Confessions of a
Con Man," 1909; "Warrior, the Untamed,"
1909; "The House of Mystery," 1910; "The
Readjustment," 1910; "The Red Button," 1912;
"Where the Heart is," 1912; "Beating Back"
(with Al. J. Jennings), 1914; "Men, Women and
War," 1915; "The Latin at War," 1916; "A
Reporter in Armageddon," 1918; "The Thir-
teenth Chair" (a play with Bayard Veilers) 1916;
"The Next War," 1921; "Columbine Time,"
1921; "Christ or Mars," 1921; "Youth Rides
West," 1925. He is author, also, of the follow-
ing pamphlets: "The Babes of Belgium;" "The
Splendid Story of Ypres," 1915.

Mr. Irwin is nearly fifty-two years old and is
much more vigorous than most men of his age.
He lives in New York, where he owns a home in
Greenwich Village, but spends his summers in

Scituate, Massachusetts. At the present time, he is writing fiction, having just published that splendid novel, "Youth Rides West," in which he tells of his experiences in the mining camp of his boyhood days.

The work which Mr. Irwin has accomplished may to some seem almost incredible, but it shows what success one may achieve, subsequent to an attack of pulmonary tuberculosis.

ALBERT EDWARD WIGGAM

A LBERT EDWARD WIGGAM was born
on a farm near Austin, in southern
Indiana, on the day the Chicago fire
broke out, October 9, 1871. His mother and
father died before he reached the age of nine
and he was reared by a stepmother on a farm
at Deputy, Indiana, until he was twelve and,
later, at Vernon, Indiana, where he still makes
his summer home in the old family homestead.
He credits not only his education, but his life,
to the care, affection and foresight of this wonderful woman who reared him with his seven
brothers and sisters, kept them together, and
conserved the moderate means left by his father
for the education of the children. At fourteen,
after a summer in a country academy, he went
for a year to Moore's Hill College, Indiana, and
then, later, to Hanover College, where he
graduated at the age of twenty-one, having been
delayed in his progress for two years by ill
health, due to an attack of malarial fever. He
really completed the four years of the regular
college work in three and a half years, taking
both the classical and scientific courses. Partly

to earn money for his further education and partly to explore the country, he had left college for one year and had sold books throughout the southern states. This year of hard contacts with his fellow men, of training in the arts of salesmanship, and of learning to hold the interest of people, Mr. Wiggam counts the most valuable single period of his educational development.

After graduating from Hanover, he packed his trunk and started for Johns Hopkins University where he planned to take a Doctor's degree in Political Science. He got as far as Cincinnati, where physicians told him he had advanced pulmonary tuberculosis. He had been active in athletics, and especially in tennis, and he was fond of hunting; but he had suffered a number of hemorrhages during his last year in college. This diagnosis ended his formal scholastic career. He went the following autumn to Colorado where, for five years, he lived the usual life of the "lunger," out of a job most of the time, and badly discouraged over the seeming waste of his years. During this time he knocked about, spending one winter in Colorado College taking lectures in Philosophy. Later he became an assayer of silver and gold and, in company with a mining and civil engineer, laid out a mining camp for a large eastern company.

By this time, he felt confident enough of his health to go East and proceeded as far as Minneapolis where he secured a position as a newspaper reporter on the *Minneapolis Journal.* He was better fitted for editorial writing so he devoted most of his time to that branch for the following year.

While in Minneapolis, Mr. Wiggam developed his latent talent for public speaking. His father, although primarily a farmer, was, nevertheless, famed in southern Indiana for his oratorical gifts. A Chicago lecture bureau made Wiggam an offer, and he spent the years of 1899 and 1900 on the lecture platform. Realizing his lack of specialized or authoritative knowledge in any particular field he began to study intensively medical sociology and public health. For three years he lectured upon medical and dental inspection in the schools and aroused a great many cities and counties to take active interest in this direction. His lectures in this field became so popular that he was asked to speak before many medical societies throughout the country. He received the enthusiastic approval of the medical profession for his sanity, caution and thoroughly scientific spirit. He never lectured upon any theme without an authentic background of knowledge in the literature of his subject.

Mr. Wiggam married Elizabeth Jayne, of
North Vernon, Indiana, in 1902. Heredity
and the special phase of the inheritance of
acquired characteristics was the subject of world-
wide controversy at this time. Wiggam saw
that if this thesis was true, medical science,
instead of strengthening the race in its structural
values, was contributing to its deterioration by
its saving of the weaklings. He conceived the
idea that something far more fundamental than
a campaign for the social application of medical
science through public health measures was
necessary. In accordance with his habit he
began intensive study in this extended field.
He visited biological laboratories in this country
and in Europe. Aided by his wife he began the
collection of publications devoted to these phases
of biology. In 1909, he had the largest private
collection of the literature of heredity, genetics
and eugenics in the world. He began the
delivery of popular lectures, the first to be given
on these subjects by a professional student.

In speaking of his lecture work, he says: "I
have myself traveled many hundreds of thousands of miles over this country, lecturing. I
have lectured to audiences in universities and
small colleges; in mining and lumber camps, in
gold-leafed ball rooms; to labor conventions,

capitalists; women's clubs, men's clubs, millionaires' clubs, down-and-out clubs, and to Opie Read's "Arkansas Travelers in the Ozark."

During these years his health was in a precarious state and at times it seemed imperative that he should give up all work and take prolonged rests. In addition to his general disability, his eyes gradually weakened, until after the year 1906 he was entirely unable to read. His wife became his reading secretary and has read aloud practically everything for him since that time.

He says, "It has in some ways been a handicap and in some ways a blessing." "It has held me strictly to my specialty," he has often remarked, "and has led me to spend all my days and nights reflecting upon the facts, as well as the larger social significance of biology. It was perhaps due to this that in my many days of being blindfolded which I still often have to go through, in order to keep out the intense pain of the slightest light, my thoughts turned to the moral and ethical and spiritual meanings of science to mankind. When I was a boy I got a Sunday School paper which said that it was wicked to have a headache. That thought impressed me all my life. The most impressive thing about science to me was its technical meanings and its enormous effectiveness in giving men new powers to coöperate with each other and with the universe, which seemed to me to be what men call righteousness. And this thought widened with me until I was asked some years ago to write an essay for the *Century Magazine* on the ethical meaning of science. When I came home Mrs. Wiggam, at the supper table, asked me why I did not merely take the advertisement for one of my lectures and make it into a short magazine article. I did so and wrote 'The New Decalogue of Science' before I went to bed and never changed it afterward. It went all over the world and was translated into several foreign languages. It took me months, with the aid of a secretary, to answer the resulting correspondence and, especially, the kind letters from scientific men in this country and Europe. Later the publisher asked me to enlarge it into a book. I told them it could not be done, as I had said all there was to say. But after reflecting a couple of days, I saw the entire book and wrote it in sixty days. Whether good or bad, that is the way my first book was written."

In speaking of "The New Decalogue of Science," the renowned sociologist of Columbia University, Professor Franklin Giddings, says that it is "The most important contribution to popular education that has been made in America in fifty years."

During the war, Mr. Wiggam did service for the Red Cross in France. After the war, when delivering a lecture on heredity, a magazine editor chanced to hear him and asked him to write some articles on the subject. He is now officially connected with a number of magazines and is a member of the editorial staff of *The American Magazine*. In addition, he frequently writes Sunday articles for a newspaper syndicate. His magazine contributions on heredity were collected and published, under the title of "The Fruit of the Family Tree," which became a "best seller," as the Decalogue had been.

In 1923, owing to a long period of strenuous writing, he took another four months' rest because of a fresh outbreak of tuberculosis. "I knew I was going to have to," he said, "but I believed I knew about how far to go 'before taking the count.' If every one would just lie down right where he is the moment the symptoms show up and take absolute, scientific rest, he is well nigh sure to make the riffle. But if you go even six weeks too long, you may have a hard prolonged struggle. I have the utmost respect for tuberculosis, but I haven't the slightest fear of it. If a fellow will just lay off *in time* and make his rest *absolute*, the chances are all in his favor. I wanted to be a doctor, but I knew I would never stand up under the strain of being the kind of doctor I wanted to be. So maybe I have done the next best thing,—tried to make the biological sciences interesting and helpful to the common man."

In *The American Magazine*, of July, 1925, appeared an article by Mr. Wiggam under the caption of "The Ten Marks of an Educated Man." If this article could only be placed in the hands of, and be read by every American citizen, the cause of education in the entire nation would be greatly lifted. It would develop a better understanding between the people who have profited by educational advantages and those who have not had such advantages. His "ten marks" are so excellent that I cannot refrain from quoting them here.

1. He keeps his mind open on every question until the evidence is all in.
2. He always listens to the man who knows.
3. He never laughs at new ideas.
4. He cross-examines his day-dreams.
5. He knows his strong point and plays it.

6. He knows the value of good habits and how to form them.
7. He knows when not to think, and when to call in the expert to think for him.
8. You can't sell him magic.
9. He lives the forward-looking, outward-looking life.
10. He cultivates a love of the beautiful.

The following is a brief extract of the editorial comments which appeared with these "ten marks":

"Many people still cling to what one prominent college dean has called the 'camel theory' of education. They think that, as a camel can prepare for a long journey across the arid desert by drinking large quantities of water, so they themselves can fill their minds with knowledge in their youth and 'live off it' for the rest of their natural life.

"Education, however, is much more than a supply of knowledge. It is, first of all, as Mr. Wiggam points out, a state of mind and spirit, a yearning to know the truth, and a courage great enough to act upon the truth once it is known.

"So the college man is not the only one who has the chance to become educated. A man, unlearned in book lore, as Mr. Wiggam explains, may be profoundly educated. Perhaps his fund of knowledge along formal lines may not be great, but he may be great in wisdom, tolerance, and open-mindedness. Such a man is better educated than the best informed man in the world, provided that the latter has a sealed mind.

"If you have attended college, or even high school, you can, if you will make the effort, become an educated man or woman. Mr. Wiggam points out the way. He shows you the true education, which is rich in poise, power and freedom. It is open to all."

In addition to all his work in biology and in closely allied subjects, through his lectures and his publications, Mr. Wiggam is contributing a real and lasting service in the fight against disease. He is thoroughly cognizant of the fact that rest is our greatest aid in fighting tuberculosis. He says: "I feel that our growing knowledge of the value of rest is the greatest thing we have to offer the patient." He has also become greatly interested in the value of sunshine in the treatment of disease. In fact, he has an outdoor-air-dome in his back-yard where he frequently takes sunbaths as a general tonic. He is also very much interested in the problem of a window glass that will admit ultra-violet rays. When this is available, he plans to build a bungalow for winter use on the top of one of New York's apartment buildings, just because he wants "to live long and happily and healthily."

At the age of fifty-three years, Mr. Wiggam is in excellent health. He plays nine holes of golf every day and does a tremendous amount of work. What a pity that such a valuable man should have been lost to the medical profession because of tuberculosis! But *was* he lost to the medical profession? Although his health did not permit him to take a medical degree, he completed three years of study; and who, in the medical profession is doing more than he to educate the public and to create the right attitude on the part of the public toward the development of scientific truth? He lectures even before such medical groups as the Clinical Staff of the Mayo Clinic. After all, one wonders if he has not already contributed a greater service to the world through the development of his broad views of science and the translation of our scientific language into the terms of the general public than he could possibly have contributed in the practice of medicine. Be that as it may,

ALBERT EDWARD WIGGAM

Mr. Wiggam is an outstanding example of one who has suffered from tuberculosis, has overcome it, and has done and is doing a service to humanity which the world can never forget.

REFERENCES

The Ten Marks of An Educated Man. By A. E. Wiggam. *The American Magazine*, July, 1925.

EUGENE O'NEILL

EUGENE O'NEILL was born in the old Barrett House, Forty-third and Broadway, New York City, on October 16, 1888. He is the son of James O'Neill, the famous actor of a generation ago. His parents spent most of their time traveling and Eugene was with them until the age of seven years when the parents decided to enroll him in a convent school. Sometime after this he was sent to a preparatory school and when he was eighteen years old he entered Princeton University. He did not enjoy college life, nor was he amenable to the discipline, so after one year he was suspended. It was understood that at the end of that year Eugene might return, but he did not care to return. Instead he secured a position with a small mail order firm, but after one year he, as well as the firm, were more than ready for his departure. Then he went to Honduras to prospect for gold, but after six months he developed a fever and was sent home without gold. Next he secured the assistant managership of the company in which his father was playing. Although he had a great dislike for this kind of work, he continued in it for six months. Later he went to sea aboard a Norwegian bark, on a voyage that lasted sixty-five days. When he landed at Buenos Aires he secured positions with such companies as the Swift Packing Company, the Westinghouse Company, and the Singer Sewing Machine Company, but each of these positions was held only for a short time. From Buenos Aires he sailed to Portuguese, South Africa, and thence back to New York.

O'Neill relates some of his experiences there as follows: "In New York, I lived at 'Jimmy the Priest's', a waterfront dive, with a back room where you could sleep with your head on the table if you bought a schooner of beer. 'Jimmy the Priest's' place is the original of the saloon in 'Anna Christie.' And an old sailor whom I knew there is the original of 'Chris,' the father in the play.

"Again I hung around the waterfront for a while. There, as at Buenos Aires, I picked up an occasional job aboard a vessel that was loading or unloading. The work was mostly cleaning ship; painting, washing the decks, and so on.

"After a few weeks, or months, I shipped on the American Liner *New York*, as an able seaman. I made the voyage to Southampton; and as the

New York was disabled, I came back on the *Philadelphia*. But there was about as much 'sea glamour' in working aboard a passenger steamship as there would have been in working in a summer hotel! I washed enough deck area to cover a good-sized town.

"It was on these two voyages that I got to know the stokers, although it did not really begin aboard ship. There is class distinction even among the groups that make up the crew of an ocean liner. But in this case, one group does not regard another as superior to it. Each has a healthy contempt for the others.

"I shouldn't have known the stokers if I hadn't happened to scrape an acquaintance with one of our own furnace-room gang at 'Jimmy the Priest's.' His name was Driscoll, and he was a Liverpool Irishman. It seems that years ago some Irish families settled in Liverpool. Most of them followed the sea, and they were a hard lot. To sailors all over the world, a 'Liverpool Irishman' is the synonym for a tough customer. It was through Driscoll that I got to know other stokers, Driscoll himself coming to a strange end. He committed suicide by jumping overboard in midocean. . . ."

From New York O'Neill went to New Orleans. Here he learned from a theater advertisement

that his father was in the city playing an engagement. Through his father's persuasion O'Neill
took one of the minor parts in the play. Later
with his parents he returned to New London,
Connecticut, where he became a local newspaper
reporter.

During this period, through his adventures as
a denizen of the docks, a friend of gamblers,
stoker and Tammany Hall politician, newspaper
reporter and actor, he contracted tuberculosis.
He was twenty-five years of age when he
entered Gaylord Farm Sanatorium. Dr. David
Lyman, one of America's most favorably known
tuberculosis workers, was superintendent of the
Gaylord Farm Sanatorium where O'Neill was
advised to go. Dr. Lyman not only has worked
with such physicians as E. L. Trudeau and
Lawrason Brown and is unexcelled in tuberculosis work, but also possesses that great spirit of
kindness and helpfulness which radiates to all
with whom he comes in contact. Up to this
time O'Neill had pursued no definite plan in
life, but his stay in the sanatorium completely
changed his outlook.

He wrote some poetry in the sanatorium, and
explains his reactions to the institution thus:
"No, it isn't exactly true that my first urge to
write came at the San. Previous to my break-

down I had done quite a lot of newspaper work in New London which included original poems, parodies, verses, etc., for the editorial page, and this experience started me, although the work itself was junk of the low order. But it was at Gaylord that my mind got the chance to establish itself, to digest and valuate the impressions of many past years in which one experience had crowded on another with never a second's reflection. At Gaylord I really *thought* about my life for the first time, about past and future. Undoubtedly the inactivity forced upon me by the life at a san forced me to mental activity, especially as I had always been highstrung and nervous temperamentally."

The first year after leaving the sanatorium he wrote eleven one-act plays and two long plays. His life of adventure and his inside experiences have given him the poise, severe judgment and deliberateness of speech that have made him "The American Playwright." A year at Harvard was spent under Professor Baker perfecting his technique of the drama.

O'Neill had difficulty in securing a publisher, an experience that is not unusual with writers before their reputation is established. He explains the long interval between the writing of his plays and their publication as follows: "I sent two of the plays to a well-known New York manager. After two years, having heard nothing from them, I wrote asking for their return. They came back to me in the original package in which I had sent them. They hadn't even been read.

"Another time, I asked my father, who was a personal friend of George Tyler, to send two of my plays to him. I thought a little influence might at least get them read. Mr. Tyler's firm failed a year or two later, but it wasn't due to my plays. For when the affairs of the firm were settled up the 'scripts were returned to me; and again they were unread.

"Tyler told me afterward that when they came to him, with a letter from my father, he said to himself, 'Oh! So Jim O'Neill's son has been writing some plays. Well, they can't be any good, because plays by actors' sons are never good!' And he put them away in a drawer and didn't even look at them.

"The first recognition of any kind that I received was from *The Smart Set*. I sent three of my one-act plays to Mencken, the editor. They were all three 'fo'c'cle' plays, not at all the kind of thing *The Smart Set* prints. I wrote Mencken that I knew this, but that I merely wanted his opinion of them. I had a fine letter from him, saying that he liked them and was sending them to George Jean Nathan, the dramatic critic. I received a letter from Nathan also, and to my surprise the three plays were published in *The Smart Set!* That was my first ray of recognition.

"Then, one summer I came to Provincetown, and here I met the group that had organized under the name of Provincetown Players. They had a little theater in an old building on one of the wharves. It's rather a curious coincidence that my first production should have been on a wharf in a sea town. The piece itself was 'Bound East for Cardiff.' The scene was laid on shipboard; and while it was being acted you could hear the waves washing in and out under the wharf."

Upon being asked how he gets the idea and works out a play he gave the following reply: "Oh, the idea usually begins in a small way. I may have it sort of hanging around in my mind for a long time before it grows into anything definite enough to work on. The idea for 'The Emperor Jones' was in my mind for two years before I wrote the play. I never try to force an idea. I think about it off and on. If nothing seems to come of it, I put it away and forget it. But apparently my subconscious mind keeps working on it; for, all of a sudden, some day, it comes back to my conscious mind as a pretty well formed scheme.

"When I finally get to work I write the whole play out in long hand. Then I go over it, and rewrite it in long hand. Then I type it, making a good many changes as I go along. After that, I like to put it away for a few months, if possible; then take it out and go over it again. There wasn't any difficulty in doing this until recently. When I began writing, I would have put my plays away for a few years, without anyone knowing or caring. It is getting to be different now."

Even though O'Neill has accomplished a great deal in the literary field he has kept a careful watch over his health. He says: "After I left the san, I kept up the sleeping outdoors for over a year and kept pretty careful watch over myself generally. In fact, with more or less frequent lapses due to rehearsals in New York, etc., I've lived a pretty healthy outdoor life, ever since. It's easy, for I much prefer it to city life, anyway."

"The Straw," written from O'Neill's experiences, has a unique appeal since the setting is laid in a sanatorium and the reactions of Eileen Carmody to her environment are typical. This is the only drama in English that deals intimately with sanatorium life.

At one time when asked about his scheme of life, or his philosophy, he said: "Well, I suppose it is the idea I try to put into all of my plays. People talk of the 'tragedy' in them, and call it 'sordid,' 'depressing,' 'pessimistic'—the words usually applied to anything of a tragic nature. But tragedy, I think, has the meaning the Greeks gave it. To them it brought exaltation, an urge toward deeper spiritual understandings and released them from the petty greeds of every-day existence. When they saw a tragedy on the stage they felt their own hopeless hopes ennobled in art.

"Any victory we may win is never the one we dreamed of winning. The point is that life in itself is nothing. It is the dream that keeps us fighting, willing, living! Achievement, in the narrow sense of possession, is a stale finale. The dreams that can be completely realized are not worth dreaming. The higher the dream, the more impossible it is to realize it fully. But you would not say, since this is true, that we should dream only of easily attained ideals. A man wills his own defeat when he pursues the unattainable. But his struggle is his success! He is an example of the spiritual significance which life attains when it aims high enough, when the individual fights all the hostile forces within and without himself to achieve a future of nobler values.

"Such a figure is necessarily tragic. But to me he is not depressing; he is exhilarating! He may be a failure in our materialistic sense. His treasures are in other kingdoms. Yet isn't he the most inspiring of all successes?

"If a person is to get the meaning of life he must 'learn to like' the facts about himself— ugly as they may seem to his sentimental vanity—before he can lay hold on the truth behind the facts; and that truth is never ugly!"

In writing of O'Neill's life at present, Mary B. Mullett said: "I went to see him recently at his summer home, though he sometimes stays there as late as November. The house, until a few years ago, was the Peeked Hill Bars Coast Guard Station, on the dunes a few miles from Provincetown, Massachusetts. From it, not another house is to be seen. The only human habitations are the new station, a quarter of a mile away, and a small shack. But these are hidden by the hills of sand.

"It is a desolation of sand and sea; but very beautiful—also very remote! Few persons could plow through the soft sand to reach it, fewer

[315]

still would do so. An automobile would be
'mired' in sand within a few feet. Only a horse
can make the trip.

"From June until late in the autumn, O'Neill
lives and works there. The household consists
of himself, his wife, their three-year-old son, a
housekeeper, and the child's nurse.

"And here is an interesting fact: O'Neill has
a regular habit of work. The craving for freedom, for the indulgence of his own desires,
which controlled him in his early manhood, is
subordinated now to the good of his work. He,
who used to be a rebel against routine, volun-
tarily follows a routine now, in this one direction.
Like the rest of us, he has found that he must
follow a regular habit of work if he is to accomplish anything."

O'Neill firmly believes that sanatorium treatment taken in the right spirit, changes one for
the better. In this connection he says: "I'm
sure it did me, and the harder the patient's fight
has been, the more this applies, I should think.
After having conquered T.B. by a long grind of
struggles, one's confidence in coming out on top
in other battles ought to be increased ten-fold."

His message to tuberculous patients is: "My
only message (and I feel it's rather impertinent
for one like me, who had to fight so little, to give

a 'message' to those who may have a real man-size battle on their hands) is: Win out and God bless you—And here's my loudest cheers!

"But let me add a warning: Don't get snobbish. I remember I used to sort of despise the untutored, ignorant folk who did not have or had not had T.B. I looked down upon such unfortunates as an inexperienced, inferior lot, who after all, couldn't know much about life or anything else. They simply didn't belong, thought I with a superior sniff—until one day a friend, an eminent T.B. specialist, sensing my attitude, maliciously told me that truth—that autopsies reveal the democratic fact that nearly everyone has had it! Which leaves us only one point of superiority to brag about: We know it and the rest of them don't."

O'Neill's genius has been recognized in Europe as well as in America and his popularity there is noteworthy. Like Robert Louis Stevenson, tuberculosis played a big part in his life. Ultimately he might have drifted into the literary field, but his stay in Gaylord Farm Sanatorium gave him an opportunity for retrospection. It also gave him an opportunity to plan for his future life work, leading him to a place in the front rank of American dramatists to become "the most significant playwright in America."

Thus we must record another case of a young person's life being diverted, finding itself, catching a great vision and carrying on to the realization of his vision, and more largely because of the development of tuberculosis in his own body. If the Gaylord Farm Sanatorium with its superintendent, Dr. Lyman, had the saving of just this one life to its credit, its existence throughout the past and for all future times would be more than justified. What greater accomplishment could be desired than the saving of a life that later brings to thousands, throughout the world, practical messages resulting in enlightenment and happiness of the human family. This, and more, was accomplished in saving the life and extending the years of usefulness of Eugene O'Neill.

REFERENCES

What a Sanatorium Did for Eugene O'Neill. By J. F. O'Neill. *The Journal of the Outdoor Life*, June, 1923.
The Extraordinary Story of Eugene O'Neill. By Mary B. Mullett. *The American Magazine*, November, 1922.
Eugene O'Neill, the American Playwright. By Oliver Martin Sayler.